T0224739

SpringerBriefs in Applied Sciences
and Technology

Computational Intelligence

Series Editor

Janusz Kacprzyk, Systems Research Institute, Polish Academy of Sciences,
Warsaw, Poland

SpringerBriefs in Computational Intelligence are a series of slim high-quality publications encompassing the entire spectrum of Computational Intelligence. Featuring compact volumes of 50 to 125 pages (approximately 20,000-45,000 words), Briefs are shorter than a conventional book but longer than a journal article. Thus Briefs serve as timely, concise tools for students, researchers, and professionals.

More information about this subseries at https://link.springer.com/bookseries/10618

KC Santosh · Loveleen Gaur

Artificial Intelligence and Machine Learning in Public Healthcare

Opportunities and Societal Impact

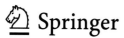 Springer

KC Santosh ⓘ
University of South Dakota
Vermillion, SD, USA

Loveleen Gaur ⓘ
Amity University
Noida, India

ISSN 2191-530X   ISSN 2191-5318 (electronic)
SpringerBriefs in Applied Sciences and Technology
ISSN 2625-3704   ISSN 2625-3712 (electronic)
SpringerBriefs in Computational Intelligence
ISBN 978-981-16-6767-1   ISBN 978-981-16-6768-8 (eBook)
https://doi.org/10.1007/978-981-16-6768-8

This Springer imprint is published by the registered company Springer Nature Singapore Pte Ltd.
The registered company address is: 152 Beach Road, #21-01/04 Gateway East, Singapore 189721, Singapore

Dedication and motivation

This book is dedicated to all the researchers, scientists, and healthcare workers who worked tirelessly to combat with COVID-19 pandemic.

The book is motivated by the following statements:

"For he who has health has hope; and he who has hope, has everything—Thomas Carlyle."

"Healthcare is vital to all of us some of the time, but public health is vital to all of us all of the time—C. Everett Koop."

"The care of public health is the first duty of the statesman—Benjamin Disraeli"

"Life's most persistent and urgent question is, 'What are you doing for others?—Martin Luther King Jr."

"So we need two things: first, we need ways of predicting and detecting disease well before it becomes life threatening; and second, we need medicines that work for you and your unique body—Pieter Cullis."

"The good or healthy society would then be defined as one that permitted people's highest purposes to emerge by satisfying all their basic needs—Abraham Maslow."

"We're at the beginning of a golden age of AI. Recent advancements have already led to invention that previously lived in the realm of science fiction—and we've only scratched the surface of what's possible—Jeff Bezos"

"Ethics is knowing the difference between what you have the right to do and what is right to do—Potter Stewart"

Foreword

I am incredibly honored and delighted to write a foreword for this highly informative and timely book *Artificial Intelligence and Machine Learning in Public Healthcare: Opportunities and Societal Impact*. As an infectious disease physician intimately involved in COVID-19, tuberculosis, and HIV-related medical care, education and research as well Director of the Mayo Clinic Center for Tuberculosis, a World Health Organization Collaborating Center In digital health and precision medicine for tuberculosis, I have real appreciation for the potential of artificial intelligence and machine learning to advance the objectives of public health. The COVID-19 pandemic has further highlighted the importance of modern ideas, fresh players, new approaches, and up-to-date technologies in understanding, preventing, forecasting, and managing diseases of public health and global importance. As difficult as coping with COVID-19 has been and continues to be, I would like to think that it has united us with a single agenda of *better health and safety globally.*

The authors have brilliantly covered opportunities, trends, concerns, and challenges associated with the incorporation of Artificial Intelligence (AI) into healthcare. The book is aimed to attract those readers who are interested in understanding the fundamental structure of AI as it relates healthcare. Healthcare professionals, medical scientists, and AI researchers in both academia and industry can benefit from this book.

In addition to describing the current landscape and future trends of AI in public health, this book will go a long way to advocate for the importance of integrating intelligent tools and techniques with public health for better and sustainable future. I heartily congratulate the authors for producing such an excellent work amidst these unprecedented difficult times.

Zelalem Temesgen, MD FIDSA
Professor of Medicine
Director
Mayo Clinic Center for Tuberculosis—A World
Health Organization—Collaborating Center in
Digital Health and Precision Medicine
Director
HIV Program, Division of Infectious Diseases
Mayo Clinic
Editor-in-Chief: Journal of Clinical Tuberculosis
and Other Mycobacterial Diseases

Preface

Public health requires special attention as it drives economy and education system. COVID-19 is an example—a truly infectious disease outbreak. The vision of WHO is to create public health services that can deal with above-mentioned crucial challenges by focusing on the following elements: health protection, disease prevention, and health promotion. For these issues, in the big data analytics era, AI-driven and Machine Learning (ML) tools and/or techniques have potential to improve public health (e.g. existing healthcare solutions and wellness services). In other words, they have proved to be valuable tools not only to analyze/diagnose pathology but also to accelerate decision-making procedure especially when we consider resource-constrained regions. This book discusses and evaluates actual and potential contributions with AI and ML algorithms in dealing with challenges that are primarily related to public health. It also helps find ways in which we can measure possible consequences and societal impacts by taking the following factors into account: open public health issues and common AI solutions (with multiple case studies such as TB and COVID-19), AI in sustainable healthcare, AI in precision medicine, and data privacy issues.

Vermillion, USA   KC Santosh
Noida, India   Loveleen Gaur

Summary

The book opens with an introduction to Artificial Intelligence (AI) in public health (Chap. 1). AI potential in reshaping healthcare is very promising, especially in resource-poor settings. It has the potential to revolutionize humankind's transformation. From drug discovery to public health, health innovation is being rolled on its head by AI. The subfields of AI, such as computer vision, surpass practitioners in accurate diagnosis in few areas; brain signals translation guides to breakthrough in recovering lost physical capacities such as speech due to stroke or other neurological conditions. Deep learning has pioneering applications in pharma and medicine, ranging from disease diagnosis to epidemic prediction. The core concept, "Transfer learning- a process that uses general datasets to create learning to specific problems", has accelerated the process of innovation. AI in public health dominates the global discussion on various dimensions ranging from future employment, economic performance, and societal change. With AI becoming an increasingly effective means to automate learning, it creates curiosity; how can society better shape AI for public value? What are the implications for patients, healthcare systems, and the community? Chap. 1 covers the well-known use cases, perks, perils, and AI challenges in transforming human society.

Chapter 2 discusses on open public health issues. Public health is an important issue that involves a substantial segment of a certain population with diseases, such as Type II diabetes, infectious diseases (e.g. Tuberculosis (TB), COVID-19, etc.), mental health challenges, and motor vehicle accidents. Unlike the healthcare field, public health is further concerned about safeguarding the entire population. The focus of public health is to slash health inequalities. The fundamental concepts are to protect the public from contagious diseases, enhance service facilities, and elevate the population's health by a healthy lifestyle. Despite the rapid evolution and advancement of medical treatments and technologies, many public health problems vexing technologically advanced nations worldwide. Overall, Chap. 2 discusses prominent global health issues and illustrates the effect from the COVID-19 pandemic perspective. The chapter will further focus on significant threats to global public health during the worldwide pandemic.

Chapter 3 discusses on possible AI solutions to public health issues/problems. Statistics and ML set the base for AI; presently, radical advances are ongoing in deep neural networks. It has established great interest in science, medicine, and public health disciplines. Researchers demonstrated that DL could accomplish alongside the finest human clinicians in precise diagnostic tasks. There is an upsurge in innovative individual health examining via mobiles and net-based communications. AI-driven health-oriented apps are now employed on handheld devices such as smartphones. The prospective impact of AI for health is majorly influenced by existing societal aspects. The past decade displayed the general diffusion of AI into health industries which has been eased by overall developments in computation power,machine processes along with congregation of health-related data due to EMRs, and health data tracking devices (e.g. smartphones, digital images, and genomic data). Chapter 3 considers the influence of AI for better future of public health, community health, and healthcare delivery. It will further be concentrated on technical competencies, applications, and limitations.

Chapter 4 includes whether AI could help build sustainable public healthcare. Sustainability and public health are deeply correlated, and public health represents a prerequisite for sustainable development of healthcare, which should be unceasingly invested in and enhanced. According to WHO, approximately 12.9 million healthcare workers will be scarce globally by 2035. In addition, around half of the world's population wants access to primary healthcare. About a hundred million people will be needy because of healthcare expenditure in chronic non-communicable diseases such as cancers, cardiovascular diseases, and diabetes.Incidentally, AI is perceived as a technology that can decrease global health disparities.Chapter 4 aims to discuss the prospective benefits of AI-based health, perils, and challenges.Further, we will delve into making the path for a responsible, sustainable, and broad use of AI.Additionally, we will ponder into question: how we can boost innovation and investment to augment well-being, health outcomes, decrease the growth of cost, and reinforce customer satisfaction.

Chapter 5 deals with AI in precision medicine. The conjunction of AI and precision medicine pledges to transform healthcare. Precision medicine intends to customize care for individuals.The practice recognizes characteristics of patients with less common reactions to medication.The objective necessitates gaining access to substantial volumes of data. The substantial advancements in medical care are precision medicine for recent years, which influences future development in the symptom-driven medical procedure. AI leverages advanced computation and conjecture to produce understandings, empowers the system to think and discover, and enables clinician decision-making through supplemented intelligence. The integration of precision medicine into healthcare can generate accurate diagnoses, predict disease probability before symptoms appear, and healthcare professionals may offer personalized medication and enhance the efficiency and safety of individuals. With the exponential rise of disruptive technologies, the growth of biomedical data is increasing rapidly, such as genome sequencing data; medical images; and drug perturbation data of healthy, developing, and diseased tissue. Various state-of-the-art technologies aim to learn from these data to understand healthy baselines and disease signatures. The application of deep learning technologies includes digital image recognition, single-cell clustering, and virtual drug screens, exhibiting the extents and dominion of AI in biomedicine. Overall, Chap. 5 aims at critically evaluating the potential of AI and its subfields in precision medicine. Further, to showcase progress in this endeavour, exemplify future needs and trends, and identify any essential prerequisites of AI and ML for precision health.

Chapter 6 includes societal impact due to AI in public healthcare. The value that technology generates for the planet is worth the risk. AI is monumental in transforming public healthcare with many innovations from drug discovery to healthcare delivery and is projected as a change-maker in healthcare. Apart from private healthcare, AI is speedily substituting traditional public healthcare systems to make enhanced healthcare accessible worldwide. With the increased integration of data-driven applications in our daily lives, anxiety is rising among individuals about the technologies' capability to disrupt their survival. Though the technical advances of AI in healthcare are tremendous, its use and social influence have fascinated various stakeholders from government to society. Overall, Chap. 6 concentrates on concerns influencing the societal impact of AI. The main concerns are bias, prejudice,confidentiality, secrecy, explainability, interpretability, societal problems, ethics, and legislation. Beyond the hype of AI in public health, let us consider the following open issues:possible technological threats, trust in AI, societal changes (with AI), information/data security, and data sharing and privacy concerns.

Chapter 7 covers case studies with a primary focus on AI for infectious diseases. Infectious diseases are a prominent reason for morbidity and mortality in individuals worldwide. However, with the evolution of industrialization after World War II, there is an upsurge in the progress of chemotherapeutic agents, an extension of public health practices, and profound innovations in microbiology and immunology, leading to substantial reductions in the prevalence of mortality and morbidity owing to infectious diseases. Researchers and healthcare specialists keep exploring new knowledge to assist in confronting virulent diseases through the latest worldwide urgency. The various studies demonstrated AI as a promising technology in a better scaleup, speed-up processing capacity, consistency, and outpace human beings in certain healthcare activities. Thus, the healthcare sector utilized several AI technologies to combat infectious diseases such as TB and COVID-19. Overall, Chap. 7 aspires to exhaustively evaluate the position of AI as a powerful technique in diagnosing,forecasting, predicting, tracking, and drug development for infectious diseases and their associated pandemic.

Chapter 8 discusses three important terms: privacy, security, and ethical issues. It seems like the blink of an eye, declaring the pervasive presence of AI in the healthcare industry. However, AI is at the peak of its hype curve, and it is also facing critique from its cynics and passion from die-hard evangelists. Economic forecasters have forecasted fiery progress in AI-driven healthcare in the future times. With this exponential growth arises several challenges. It is necessary to explore the privacy, security, and ethical aspects of AI systems to prevent inadvertent, adverse after-effects and perils occurring from the operation of AI in healthcare. Briefly, Chap. 8 maps the privacy, security, and ethical challenges posed by AI in healthcare and recommends ways for resolving them, particularly emphasizes the significance of developing an AI-driven healthcare system that is effective and fosters confidence.

Keywords: Artificial intelligence, machine learning, deep learning, public healthcare, precision medicine, sustainable healthcare, infectious disease, data privacy, security, ethical issues, societal impact.

Contents

About the Authors

Prof. KC Santosh, Ph.D. is Chair of the Department of Computer Science at the University of South Dakota (USD). He also serves International Medical University as an Adjunct Professor (Full). Before joining USD, he worked as Research Fellow at the US National Library of Medicine (NLM), National Institutes of Health (NIH). He was Postdoctoral Research Scientist at the Loria Research Centre (with industrial partner, ITESOFT (France)). He has demonstrated expertise in artificial intelligence, machine learning, pattern recognition, computer vision, image processing, and data mining with applications- such as medical imaging informatics, document imaging, biometrics, forensics and speech analysis. His research projects are funded (of more than $2m) by multiple agencies, such as SDCRGP, Department of Education, National Science Foundation, and Asian Office of Aerospace Research and Development. He is the proud recipient of the Cutler Award for Teaching and Research Excellence (USD, 2021), the President's Research Excellence Award (USD, 2019), and the Ignite from the U.S. Department of Health & Human Services (2014). For more info. follow http://kc-santosh.org.

Prof. Loveleen Gaur, Ph.D. is Professor and Program Director, Artificial Intelligence & Business Intelligence and Data Analytics of the Amity International Business School, Amity University, Noida, India. She is Senior IEEE Member and Series Editor with CRC and Wiley. She has significantly contributed to enhancing scientific understanding by participating in over three hundred scientific conferences, symposia, and seminars, by chairing technical sessions and delivering plenary and invited talks. She has specialized in the fields of artificial intelligence, machine learning, pattern recognition, Internet of things, data analytics, and business intelligence. She has chaired various positions in the international conferences of repute and is Reviewer with top-rated journals of IEEE, SCI, and ABDC Journals. She has been honored with prestigious national and international awards. She is also actively involved in various reputed projects of Government of India and abroad.

Acronyms

AF	Atrial Fibrillation
AI	Artificial Intelligence
ARIMA	Autoregressive Integrated Moving Average
BERT	Bidirectional Encoder Representations from Transformer
CAD	Computer-Aided Diagnosis
CAGR	Compound Annual Growth Rate
CNN	Convolution Neural Network
COPD	Chronic Obstructive Pulmonary Disease
CT	Computed Tomography
CXR	Chest X-ray
DL	Deep Learning
DNA	Deoxyribonucleic acid
ECG	Electrocardiogram
EMR	Electronic Medical Record
FDA	Food and Drug Administration
GPS	Global Positioning System
HIPAA	Health Insurance Portability and Accountability Act
HIV	Human Immunodeficiency Virus
IBM	International Business Machines
ICD	International Classification of Diseases
ICU	Intensive Care Unit
ISO	International Organization for Standardization
LSTM	Long Short-term Memory
MDG	Millennium Development Goal
ML	Machine Learning
MRI	Magnetic Resonance Image
NCD	Non-communicable Disease
NGS	Next-Generation Sequencing
NLP	Natural Language Processing
NTD	Neglected Tropical Disease
OCR	Optical Character Recognition

PACS	Picture Archiving and Communication System
PET	Positron Emission Tomography
RF	Random Forest
RNA	Ribonucleic Acid
RNN	Recurrent Neural Network
SARS	Severe Acute Respiratory Syndrome
SVM	Support Vector Machine
TB	Tuberculosis
UHC	Universal health coverage
UNSDG	United Nation Sustainability Development Goal
US	United States
WHO	World Health Organization
XAI	Explainable AI

List of Figures

List of Tables

Chapter 1
Introduction to AI in Public Health

1.1 Introduction

AI began as a series of "if–then rules" and has advanced over several decades to include more complex algorithms surpassing human brains. AI has rapidly evolved and is ubiquitous from language differentiation, image processing, handwriting detection, weather forecasting, and search engines. It brings a transformation to healthcare, driven by massive and increasingly available healthcare data and accelerated AI techniques growth.

Broadly, AI techniques are classified into three categories: (a) traditional Machine Learning (ML), (b) advanced Deep Learning (DL), and (c) Natural Processing Language (NLP). Many AI applications in medicine and health, ranging from chronic diseases to radiology and risk assessment, where AI techniques can have impactful interventions [1].

The data is regularly produced from clinical pursuits and physical examination documents, and medical imaging, both in a structured and unstructured formats. AI techniques can be applied to both forms of data. ML, the classification of AI techniques, is majorly used to classify and predict structured data. Natural Language Processing (NLP), another type of AI technique, is deployed to analyze unstructured (textual/handwritten) data. The fast growth in NLP has yielded AI systems with significant abilities that have vastly impacted the economy. Fortune 500 companies like Google and Microsoft have installed the Bidirectional Encoder Representations from Transformers (BERT) language model into their search engines [2, 3].

Deep Learning (DL), a novel extension of ML, is widely popular and applicable in analyzing complex patterns from vast volumes of complex data (e.g. medical images). DL variants such as convolution neural networks (CNN) and recurrent neural networks (RNN) can analyze high-dimensional data widely adopted in medical applications.

The following sections will discuss the role of AI in public health, various AI applications in healthcare, and its pros and cons.

K. Santosh and L. Gaur, *Artificial Intelligence and Machine Learning in Public Healthcare*, SpringerBriefs in Computational Intelligence, https://doi.org/10.1007/978-981-16-6768-8_1

1.2   Role of AI

According to the report of grand view research in Fig. 1.1, the size of market is evaluated at 6.7 billion (USD) in 2020 and is anticipated to grow at CAGR of 41.8% in coming years [4].

According to WHO "health is a state of complete physical, mental and social well-being than the mere absence of disease", this bold-faced definition prompts people to look beyond diseases and focus on the physical, mental, and public well-being of people. They describe public health as "science and art of prolonged life, preventing disease and promoting health to society's organized efforts". Public health has significantly impacted populations' health by making people healthy and saving lives [5, 6].

The quality of public health depends on various factors: specific geography, processes, and public health caregivers' motivation level. Due to COVID-19 virus, the demand to deploy AI techniques to achieve public health outcomes has rapidly increased. AI/ML is anticipated as a change-maker for healthcare; it has already revolutionized healthcare from diagnosis to worker productivity [7–9].

The increasing popularity of AI in public health is due to its potential to obtain significant patterns from high-dimensional datasets that may be used in early detection and diagnosis, treatment, and predicting outcomes in many clinical scenarios. Health data generated is leveraged for assisting clinicians in quick decision-making and projecting the patterns. Moreover, the most recent applications noted were permitting population assessment for pandemic readiness and reaction [10].

1.3   Timeline of AI in Healthcare

For a better understanding, the AI timeline, its brief historical perspective, and chronological evolution are shown in Fig. 1.2.

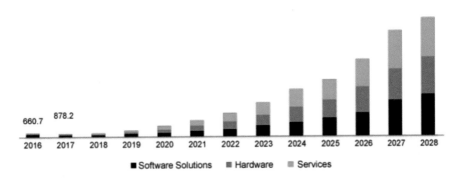

Fig. 1.1 Market size of AI in healthcare. *Source* https://www.grandviewresearch.com

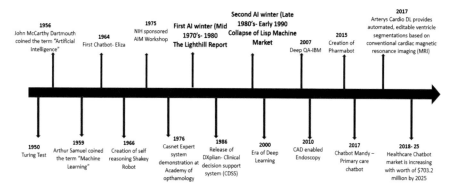

Fig. 1.2 Timeline of the advancement and usage of AI in healthcare

1.4   Use Cases of AI in Healthcare

In recent years, advancement in AI functions has been rapid, exponential, pervasive, and immersive in our lives. This section covers the few prevalent applications of AI techniques in healthcare [11].

Reducing misdiagnosis and decreasing medical inaccuracy is the vital and stimulating potential of AI application for healthcare. ML has the ability to assist pathologists in accurate diagnosis of several chronicle cancers.

- The company PathAI is developing ML technology for the prediction of cancers.
- Harvard Medical School uses Buoy health- an AI-based symptom algorithm for diagnosing and treating illness quickly.
- Enlitic builds medical tools to rationalize radiology diagnosis using images, blood examinations, genomics, and patient medical record for superior Insights.
- Freenome intends to utilize AI in general screenings, diagnoses, investigative tests, early detection of cancer, and consequently build innovative therapies.
- Beth Israel Deaconess Medical Center utilizes AI-enhanced microscopes to examine harmful bacteria in blood samples for timely identification of possibly fatal blood ailments.
- Zebra Medical Vision utilizes AI-enabled assistance to quickly analyze scans and provide support to radiologists for rapid diagnosis.

Drug development is another AI breakthrough area; biopharmaceutical enterprises are rapidly taking sight of AI algorithms' efficiency, accuracy, and knowledge [12].

- BioXcel Therapeutics utilizes AI to recognize and build new medicines in the disciplines of immuno-oncology and neuroscience. Moreover, they use AI to discover additional functions for current drugs.
- BERG-AI-based biotech company that treats rare diseases utilizing AI.

- Atomwise utilizes AI to handle severe comprising Ebola and multiple sclerosis. It facilitates the prediction of bioactivities and pinpoints patient features for clinical experiments.

AI can **enhance patient experience** by streamlining the processes and reducing delays in providing diagnosis and treatment.

- The Olive Company provides AI-as-a-service for easy and quick integration with existing tools and infrastructure and eliminating lengthy and costly integration.
- Utilizing AI, Qventus automated their existing platform by providing priority based on patient ailments. It also trails hospital waiting hours and provides details for the fastest ambulance routes.
- Babylon AI-driven chatbot notices and reviews patients' symptoms before recommending a computer-generated check-in or a confrontational visit with the doctor.

The **massive amount of healthcare data** is generated daily and needs to be streamlined and mined for getting better insights. AI again proved to be an effective technology and assisting the heath sector continue afloat with mountains of data.

- Tempus utilizes AI to filter the world's most extensive clinical and molecular databases for customized and personalized healthcare treatments.
- H2O.ai mine, systematize, and predict processes of the healthcare system. The main applications are to expect intensive care unit (ICU) transfers, enhance clinical systems, and identify a potential risk of hospital-acquired infections by patients.
- The famous IBM Watson is also helping healthcare specialists connect their data to augment hospital productivity, connect with patients, and advance treatment.
- Another well-known application, Google's DeepMind Health AI software, helps hospitals to work more efficiently by providing information about patient's ailments and suggesting treatments. It also helps track and monitor patient's health utilizing massive and comparable datasets [10, 13–15] (Fig. 1.3).

1.5   Public Health Transformation Using AI

AI has forayed into various fields and has provided a remarkable performance in health technology and public health, which is even more significant with the recent global pandemic outbreak.

Research shows the plethora of advantages of adopting AI around conventional analytics and clinical decision techniques.

- AI-powered tools provide faster diagnosis surpassing human experts, helping practitioners in high-burdened areas, and reducing diagnostics costs. The advancements in learning algorithms deliver unprecedented insights from vast and complex data in lesser time and effort, providing better diagnosis, practical treatment guidance, and efficient patient care outcomes.

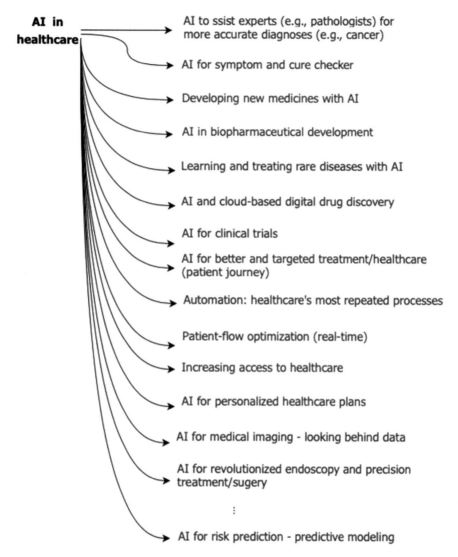

Fig. 1.3 Use cases of AI in healthcare

- AI is instrumental in reducing the burden of considerable paperwork (medical history and health records) through an AI-driven data management system, providing excellent patient care in densely populated countries. It can also help physicians provide the latest and real-time information from various repositories like medical journals, textbooks, records, clinical practices, etc., for efficient patient care.
- Along with better and accurate detection and diagnosis, AI can help identify potential risks and susceptibility of the spread of infection, which reduces the

need for human experts and reduces the burden of repeated screening in public healthcare systems.

- AI-driven apps and tools can help track health workers' productivity and monitor their day-to-day operations in densely populated and resource-poor geographies.
- They increase patient participation and awareness for successful public health campaigns, especially in population clusters (such as women and infants) where health and medical care get overlooked. The behaviour analysis and predictive analysis can help detect gaps, history of the treatment of drop out populations, and help healthcare givers provide additional counselling through awareness camps to ensure their future participation.
- NLP is widely applied to cater to the challenges of public health. Global Health Monitor, an online system and application of NLP, is used to detect and map infectious disease outbreaks. It helps to guide cancer treatments to low-resource settings. This technique mines patient health records and doctor notes for treatment advice [14–18].

1.6   Limitations of AI in Healthcare

Amidst all promises, like any other technology, AI is also not an infallible technology. It has its shortcomings as well. A few of them can be summarized as follows:

- **The generic algorithm in AI for healthcare**: Healthcare problems are care sensitive and are difficult to generalize. For example, COVID-19 and Tuberculosis (TB) are two different problems even though they come under the pulmonary abnormality category. Experts read their manifestations are read differently. It means that one AI-driven tool for both issues is merely impossible to deploy. In addition, minor changes in image pixel intensity values could easily trick AI-driven systems in the images/scans to identify benign skin lesions into malignant.
- **Inaccurate input for AI**: Slight manipulations in written descriptions of patients' conditions may also lead to different diagnoses; these small changes can readily benefit insurers and healthcare agencies.
- **Dataset**: AI extends immense gains in risk prediction and clinical decision-making procedures. The ML algorithms can only develop more specific and accurate when trained with vast amounts of data. It helps experts gain unprecedented insights into diagnosis, care practices, therapy flexibility, and patient results. In other words, AI requires a reasonably large number of datasets, which is not trivial in healthcare due to multiple confidential issues—IRB control, for example. Dealing with new disease types is always an open issue in healthcare from an AI perspective, where COVID-19 is an example [10, 13–17]. Additionally, ML scientists in the healthcare domain think of an open problem—how big data is big? [14]

Likewise, while taking payment structures into account, users/patients request extra information. AI is poised to be the tool that can build improvement throughout the care field. Do we get enough data for AI to run the game? As before, due to the lack of enough data, AI-driven tools are limited to specific problems. With such challenges in hand, all AI-driven tools do not meet commercial success [11, 19].

1.7 Challenges of AI

The section is focused on the number of challenges provided the sensitivity of health data.

Unsynchronized data structures and confidentiality constraints inside organizations and around systems restrict the volume of structured datasets that can be constructed to train algorithms.

In addition to data-related impediments, the use of ML in clinical diagnostic applications contains several inherent risks that researchers continue to struggle. A few of them are discussed below:

- Black-box decision-making is questionable and cannot be interpreted by clinicians, resulting in a misdiagnosis that is only evident after continued use.
- There is a possibility that the system is designed to make accurate decisions at the cost of either missed diagnoses or overdiagnosis. It is a predicament that human clinicians are prepared to report with conviction.
- There may be unintended consequences caused by a system trained only on ancient data or using inappropriate data points that ignore vital predictive factors, resulting in missed or inaccurate diagnoses or overdiagnosis.
- Another concern is technological, including the type of diagnostic tasks, lack of transparency of AI practice, security of AI-driven recommendations, complexities in interpreting results, and issues with AI–user interaction design.
- AI systems are, however, susceptible to hacker attacks. Hackers can alter text files or images, which may not have a human cognitive effect but could cause potentially devastating inaccuracies.
- AI triggers challenges to patient–clinician interactions, as clinicians need to realize how to interact with the AI system for healthcare delivery. Patients are required to cut the anxiety of technology.
- Ethical and trust issues are about AI and human behaviour, compatibility of machines contrasted with human value judgment, moral predicaments, and AI bias.
- AI in public health necessitates sizable datasets. Consequently, the collection, storage, and sharing of medical data raise ethical issues related to safety, governance, and privacy. Privacy is a critical concern while using AI systems because users' data (such as habits, preferences, and health records) is likely to be collected and distributed across the AI network.
- From the healthcare perspective, prejudiced AI models may overestimate or underestimate health consequences in specific patient populations. AI systems may involve labelling and display gender or racial bias. Bias in AI models may arise

when datasets are not representative of the target population or AI systems use inadequate and erroneous data for decision-making.

- Societal prejudice (such as poor access to healthcare) and trivial samples (such as minority groups) can deceive data and AI biases.

Given the challenges, there are legitimate questions about when AI technologies are suitable for patient diagnosis and treatment. Moral grey areas include using chatbots to substitute clinicians in diagnosing illnesses and permitting algorithms to triage decisions in critical care. Another debatable question is whether AI can expose patient anonymity accidentally or design fault with unintentional penalties for the use of patient records via third parties like health insurers, resulting in social bias.

To create regulations for a technology that is cloud based and perpetually advancing poses apparent challenges related to patients protection, regulatory administration, legal responsibility of stakeholders, etc. There is an urgent need for regulations and ethical standards to protect human rights and patient safety. The demand for explainable AI (XAI) is also growing to reduce the questions raised around algorithm biases. However, AI seems to retain the immense potential for altering healthcare services in resource-poor settings. There is a growing demand for these technologies to handle the challenges of public health. Future research and advancement of AI algorithms customized to resource-constrained situations will hasten AI's potential for improving global health. Coronavirus outbreak (started in December 2019)—Covid-19 is an example, where AI-guided tools can help predict (using predictive modelling) as well as diagnose/screen (using Computer-Aided Diagnosis (CAD) tools) [11, 12, 15–22].

1.8 Summary

AI has been playing an escalating and vital part globally for the past few years and impacting our daily lives. Due to pandemics, the role of AI has increased in healthcare, especially public health. No doubt, the fear of AI surpassing human abilities, yet the significant research demonstrated its wide acceptance as support in clinical decisions and enhancing treatment efficiency.

Healthcare is increasingly embracing AI-based health innovation to counter crucial health challenges. There are some significant concerns about patient privacy, legal aspects, lack of transparency, and explainability. Researchers argue that the high involvement of AI in healthcare is alarming, and the healthcare sector may gradually become money-minting business for some. There is an urgent need for regulatory bodies and policies regarding the proper usage of AI in healthcare.

For most of us, the following issues have always been open challenges:

- Ethical issues of AI in healthcare, especially for public.
- Clinical implications when integrated with ethical issues of AI in public healthcare.

- Regulatory framework for data sharing, privacy, and analysis to deploy AI-guided tools.
- Clarity in terms of AI-guided tools' limitations in public healthcare.

A growing pervasive discussion around the impending role of medical experts, specialists, and diagnosticians as AI is now ubiquitous and integrated. Will AI sooner or later take over for humans' experts? Will the forthcoming role of medical experts be squeezed into case management, screening, detection, and diagnosis to become the domain of algorithms? Will this method be adequate in the long term?

The next chapter will discuss the various open public health issues (e.g. diabetes, infectious diseases, pandemics, etc.) and global issues by health organizations.

Additional byte -◯-

Universal health coverage (UHC) implies that all entities and populations obtain the health services they want without enduring financial hardship. It comprises the complete continuum of important, quality health benefits, from health promotion to prevention, medication, rehabilitation, and relaxing care across the life path.

Source https://www.who.int/news-room/fact-sheets/detail/universal-health-coverage-(uhc).

References

1. Zhang D, Mishra S, Brynjolfsson E, Etchemendy J, Ganguli D, Grosz B, Lyons T, Manyika J, Niebles JC, Sellitto M, Shoham Y, Clark J, Perrault R (2021) The AI index 2021 annual report, AI Index Steering Committee, Human-Centered AI Institute, Stanford University, Stanford, CA, March 2021. https://aiindex.stanford.edu/wp-content/uploads/2021/03/2021-AI-Index-Report_Master.pdf
2. Benke K, Benke G (2018) Artificial intelligence and big data in public health. Int J Environ Res Public Health 15(12):2796. https://doi.org/10.3390/ijerph15122796
3. Bresnick J (2018) Top 12 ways artificial intelligence will impact healthcare. https://healthitanalytics.com/; https://healthitanalytics.com/news/top-12-ways-artificial-intelligence-will-impact-healthcare
4. Flowers J, Hall P, Pencheon D (2005) Public health indicators. Public Health 119(4):239–245. https://doi.org/10.1016/j.puhe.2005.01.003. PMID: 1573368
5. Thiébaut R, Thiessard F (2018) Artificial intelligence in public health and epidemiology. Yearb Med Inform 27(01):207–210. https://doi.org/10.1055/s-0038-1667082
6. Wahl et al (2018) Artificial intelligence (AI) and global health: how can AI contribute to health in resource-poor settings? BMJ Glob Health. https://doi.org/10.1136/bmjgh-2018-000798
7. Artificial intelligence could reshape public health, but obstacles abound NPJ Digital Medicine on Aug 16, 2019. https://www.hsph.harvard.edu/news/hsph-in-the-news/artificial-intelligence-could-reshape-public-health-but-obstacles-abound/
8. AI in public health: privacy and regulatory challenges 2020, May 09. https://www.orfonline.org/ai-in-public-health-privacy-and-regulatory-challenges-66361/
9. Yang Z, Zeng Z, Wang K, Wong SS, Liang W, Zanin M, Liu P, Cao X, Gao Z, Mai Z, Liang J, Liu X, Li S, Li Y, Ye F, Guan W, Yang Y, Li F, Luo S, Xie Y, He J (2020) Modified SEIR and AI prediction of the epidemics trend of COVID-19 in China under public health interventions. J Thorac Dis 12(3):165–174. https://doi.org/10.21037/jtd.2020.02.64

10. KC Santosh (2020) COVID-19 prediction models and unexploited data. J Med Syst 44(9):170. https://doi.org/10.1007/s10916-020-01645-z
11. Matheny M, Thadaney Israni S, Ahmed M, Whicher D (eds) (2019) Artificial intelligence in health care: the hope, the hype, the promise, the peril. NAM Special Publication. National Academy of Medicine, Washington, DC
12. Gaur L, Solanki A, Wamba SF, Jhanjhi NZ. Advanced AI techniques and applications in bioinformatics. CRC Press. https://doi.org/10.1201/9781003126164. ISBN: 978-0-367-64169-6 (hbk)
13. KC Santosh (2020) AI-driven tools for coronavirus outbreak: need of active learning and cross-population train/test models on multitudinal/multimodal data. J Med Syst 44(5):93. https://doi.org/10.1007/s10916-020-01562-1
14. KC Santosh, Ghosh S (2021) Covid-19 imaging tools: how big data is big? J Med Syst 45(7):71. https://doi.org/10.1007/s10916-021-01747-2
15. Das D, KC Santosh, Pal U (2020) Truncated inception net: COVID-19 outbreak screening using chest X-rays. Phys Eng Sci Med 43:915–925. https://doi.org/10.1007/s13246-020-00888-x
16. Mukherjee H, Ghosh S, KC Santosh (2021) Deep neural network to detect COVID-19: one architecture for both CT scans and Chest X-rays. Appl Intell 51(5):2777–2789. https://doi.org/10.1007/s10489-020-01943-6
17. Mukherjee H, Ghosh S, KC Santosh (2021) Shallow convolutional neural network for COVID-19 outbreak screening using chest X-rays. Cogn Comput. https://doi.org/10.1007/s12559-020-09775-9
18. KC Santosh (2020) COVID-19: prediction, decision-making, and its impacts. Book series in Lecture notes on data engineering and communications technologies. Springer Nature. https://doi.org/10.1007/978-981-15-9682-7
19. Joshi A, Day N, KC Santosh (2020) Intelligent systems and methods to combat COVID-19. Springer briefs in applied sciences and technology. https://doi.org/10.1007/978-981-15-6572-4. ISBN: 978-981-15-6571-7 (print), 978-981-15-6572-4 (online)
20. https://builtin.com/artificial-intelligence/artificial-intelligence-healthcare. Accessed 31 July 2021
21. Gaur L, Singh G, Agarwal V (2021) Leveraging artificial intelligence tools to combat the COVID-19 crisis. In: Singh PK, Veselov G, Vyatkin V, Pljonkin A, Dodero JM, Kumar Y (eds) Futuristic trends in network and communication technologies. FTNCT 2020. Communications in computer and information science, vol 1395. Springer, Singapore. https://doi.org/10.1007/978-981-16-1480-4_28
22. Gaur L, Bhatia U, Jhanjhi NZ et al (2021) Medical image-based detection of COVID-19 using deep convolution neural networks. Multimed Syst. https://doi.org/10.1007/s00530-021-00794-6

Chapter 2
Open Public Health Issues

2.1 Background

With globalization and increased connectivity, the effect of an incident travels across the globe with a broadband Internet connection speed. The significance of national borders is diminishing, and people and determinants of health drift liberally in every direction. World health developments pinpoint consequences of a globalized financial system, innovations in transport, and modifications to agricultural practices. It is not possible to address healthcare exclusively to local communities without taking a global view. The need to find the solution necessitates a joint attempt from people in a diversity of specialties, and global health conversation is the need of the hour [1] (Fig. 2.1).

The data demonstrate 7 of the 10 foremost reasons for fatalities in 2019 were NCDs. The globe's highest fatal disease is ischaemic heart syndrome. Stroke and pulmonary diseases are the second and third highest, respectively.

The World Bank categorizes the globe's markets into quadrants (low, lower middle, upper middle and high). The WHO global health estimates demonstrated that people staying in a low-income nation are likely to die of a contagious disease. The deaths due to ischemic heart disease and dementia happens at high-income countries (Fig. 2.2).

Global health is the awareness of healthcare from an international and interdisciplinary perspective, focusing on improving health and healthcare parity for global population. The initiatives contemplate disciplines, e.g. epidemiology, sociology, economic disparities, public policy, environmental factors, cultural studies, etc. It aims to make better public health and reinforce national security across global disease detection, active response, prevention, and control policies (Fig. 2.3).

Improving global health can enhance developed and developing countries and international security pursuits by encouraging political stability, diplomacy, and economic growth worldwide. The outbreaks of pandemics, infectious diseases, and illnesses have a significant impact on trade and travel globally. The world community

K. Santosh and L. Gaur, *Artificial Intelligence and Machine Learning in Public Healthcare*, SpringerBriefs in Computational Intelligence, https://doi.org/10.1007/978-981-16-6768-8_2

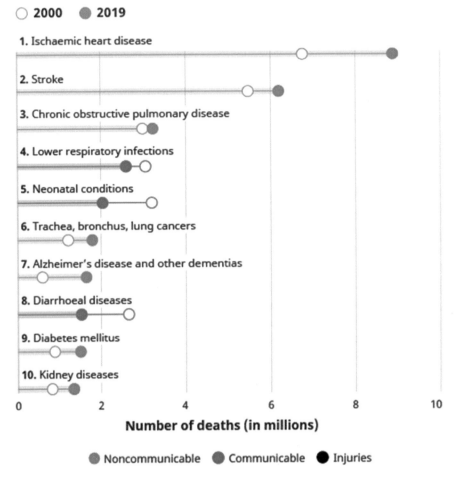

Fig. 2.1 Prominent causes of death worldwide [2]. *Source* WHO Global Health estimates. https://www.who.int/data/global-health-estimates

is discovering improved practices to tackle significant health threats by proposing new policies, guidelines and fosters teamwork among developed and developing countries on rising health concerns of global significance.

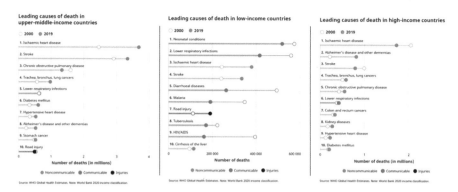

Fig. 2.2 Prominent causes of death in low-income, middle-income, and high-income countries [3]. *Source* WHO Global Health estimates: World Bank 2020 income classification https://www.who.int/data/global-health-estimates

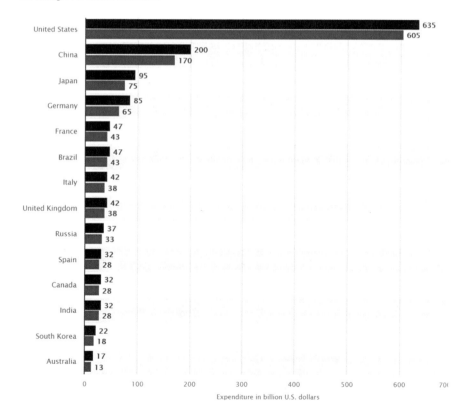

Fig. 2.3 Estimated outflow on the medicine of countries globally in 2025 (in billion U.S. dollars). *Source* https://www.statista.com/statistics/280572/medicine-spending-worldwide/

2.2 Prominent Global Health Issues

2019 brought many medical-related headlines with Chikungunya, dengue fever, and Zika epidemics [2, 4] (Table 2.1).

The year 2020 is a dreadful year for global health, laying bare the shortcomings of health systems worldwide. Moreover, it has also threatened the hard-earned progress over the past decades in fighting prominent global health issues, such as infectious diseases, mental health, disparities, and healthcare access.

WHO is confronting a plethora of challenges. Few epitomize the width and extent of this complex area:

Pandemics are epidemics with infectious disease eruptions, e.g. severe acute respiratory syndrome (SARS), Ebola, Chikungunya, Cholera, Ebola disease, Hendra infection, Influenza, Zika, Plague, HIV, and other viral diseases threats affecting substantial regions. There is no sure way to thwart the spread of disease during an outbreak, epidemic, or pandemic. These concerns are slashed off at the root level by focusing on health education, creating awareness, responsible agricultural and manufacturing practices, and the problems that trigger viruses to spread. The impact of pandemics affects the economic and social issues of countries and continents [5] (Table 2.2).

Environmental factors such as climate change and pollution are raising alarming concerns for public health. Climate change is considered the most significant danger to public health. The diseases spread more swiftly by storms, floods, droughts, pollution, and disrupt survival. Global health must prevent environmental challenges apart from providing temporary resources such as sanitation education and technology, packaged water bottles, etc. The focus should be on international policies to alleviate the human impact on climate change and environmentally conscious best practices to achieve a sustained solution [6].

Table 2.1 Countries impacted with Dengue, Chikungunya, and Zika virus (the years 2020 and 2021)

Year	Disease	Countries impacted
2020	Dengue	Bangladesh, Brazil, Cook Islands, Ecuador, India, Indonesia, Maldives, Mauritania, Mayotte (Fr), Nepal, Singapore, Sri Lanka, Sudan, Thailand, Timor-Leste, and Yemen
2021	Dengue	Brazil, Cook Islands, Colombia, Fiji, Kenya, Paraguay, Peru, and Reunion Island
2020	Chikungunya	Americas Region, Asia, and Africa
2021	Chikungunya	Americas Region, Brazil, and India
2020	Zika virus	The Caribbean, Latin America, Central Africa, India, Indonesia, Malaysia, Cambodia, and Papua New Guinea, among other places
2021	Zika virus	

Source https://www.who.int/news-room/fact-sheets/detail/dengue-and-severe-dengue

Table 2.2 Comparison of total deaths in 2019 and 2020 [1]

Cause	2019	2020
Ischaemic heart disease	8,880,000	
Stroke	6,190,000	
Chronic obstructive pulmonary disease (COPD)	3,220,000	
Lower respiratory infections	2,590,000	
Neonatal conditions	1,960,000	
COVID-19		1,800,000
Trachea, bronchus, lung cancers	1,760,000	
Alzheimer's disease and other dementias	1,590,000	
Diabetes mellitus	1,490,000	
Diarrhoeal diseases	1,450,000	

Source https://www.who.int/data/gho/data/themes/mortality-and-global-health-estimates

Healthcare disparities refer to variations in healthcare access among groups that curtail wider inequalities. These disparities occur across racial, ethnic, socio-economic status, religious conviction, age, psychological, mental, disability, sexual preference, or additional features traditionally associated with discernment or exclusion. Consequently, they confront painful experiences in sexually transmitted diseases, elevated child deaths, and nutrition.

The challenge for global health professionals is to provide equal opportunities to weaker sections or underrepresented communities in public health forums and propose policies that decrease impediments and increase access to healthcare. Parallelly encourage physicians to practice in remote areas.

Political factors Politics is a ubiquitous aspect of modern-day civilizations worldwide. Undeniably, many pathways to public health influence are political, although the precise arrangements by which these operations differ from country to country. However, there is evidence that political belief and personal benefits can put forth substantial influences on policy-making processes pertinent to health, prominent to considerable evidence–policy gaps.

Non-communicable diseases (NCDs), such as strokes, heart diseases, cancers, diabetes, chronic kidney disease, osteoarthritis, osteoporosis, Alzheimer's disease, Parkinson's disease, and cataracts, are primarily genetic, physiological, environmental, and behavioural factors. These can be prevented by providing proper education and making the population understand and change lifestyle (e.g. physical exercise, balanced diet, etc.), and discouraging toxic products (e.g. tobacco, alcohol, etc.) [2, 4, 5].

With the rise of consumption of high-fat diets and enhanced rates of smoking, strokes become prominent. There is a growth in the types of cancers that are most frequent. Based on the types of demographic and developmental evolutions expected to ensue, the WHO assesses that the deaths due to non-communicable diseases would rise to 55 million by 2030 if severe and proper actions are not taken to suppress the peril of these diseases.

Food supply and animal health are closely intertwined and one responsible factor in human health in developing countries. Poor agricultural practices such as pesticides and improper waste management may affect animal health, creating disease spread a threat to the food supply chain.

A new-found notion, i.e. "One health", intends at improving the ties between human and animal health along with the environment. The purpose is to safeguard public health through the control of pathogens in animals.

2.3 Leading Public Health Issues

Confronting key health concerns worldwide requires active involvement from various stakeholders, including government agencies, non-profit corporations, and private medical amenities. Even though the medical industry is evolving rapidly with new treatments and technologies, public health issues are plaguing worldwide and require immediate attention [7–9].

The leading public health issues for the new age are mentioned below:

- **Alcohol consumption** is a significant factor in ailment, disability, and fatality in developed countries worldwide. The health risks associated with excessive alcohol use include injuries, such as motor vehicle accidents, collapses, drownings, suicide and sexual assault, and miscarriage among pregnant women. The enduring health risks can be high blood pressure, heart disease, stroke, liver disease, digestive problems, memory problems, and mental and social health problems.
- The **human immunodeficiency virus (HIV)** is extensively contemplated as the most dangerous sexually transmitted disease (STD). It may lead to an untreatable illness, acquired immunodeficiency syndrome (AIDS), and destroys a patient's immune system. Apart from treatments, screening programs, and other public health initiatives, proper education plays a vital role in prevention, from self-restraint to appropriate use of condoms to certainly not sharing needles.
- **Heart disease and stroke** is an exceedingly preventable disease, unlike infectious diseases. Some of the well-realized risk factors include excessive tobacco use, physical inactivity, poor nutrition, and obesity. Poor heart health may consequently lead to stroke, another leading cause of death worldwide. An active lifestyle with healthy eating habits is a must for the prevention of cardiovascular diseases.
- **Prescription drug overdose happens** when a person takes more than the medically advised dose either by accidental or intentional abuse. The main reason for the quick increase in opiate violence is the marketing strategies of big pharmaceuticals companies. The primary prevention strategies are surveillance and research on drug abuse, increasing data quality and tracking developments, educating, and encouraging consumers to make healthy and safe alternatives.

Table 2.3 Facts and statistics [7]

Alcohol consumption	Three million deaths yearly, which constitutes 5.3% of all deaths
HIV	37.6 million people globally in the year 2020
Cardiovascular diseases	17.9 million lives each year (no one reason for mortality)
Opioid's overdose	0.5 million deaths
Antibiotic drug resistant	750,000 deaths yearly
Obesity	39 million children (<5 years) were overweight or obese in 2020
Foodborne illness	600 million due to contaminated food The yearly death count is 420 000

Source https://www.who.int/data/global-health-estimates

- **Antibiotic drug resistant** is becoming a big crisis for public health recently. It is ascribed to the overuse or misuse of medications. Specific bacteria/viruses can instinctively resist certain types of antibiotics and others can become resistant due to mutation in genes. The longer the duration of usage of antibiotics, the less effective they are against those bacteria. It has made treatment difficult for infectious diseases such as pneumonia, influenza, TB, and other critical illnesses such as cancers, surgery, and dialysis. Immediate steps should be taken by public health officials and doctors, such as monitoring and tracking the spread, safer practices in hospitals, stopping prescribing the overuse of antibiotics, and educating farmers about the consequences of using these antibiotics on animals (Table 2.3).
- **Lack of proper nutrition, inactivity, and obesity** are other pressing public health issues. Health officials and educators inform the general population about adopting healthy lifestyles such as avoiding fatty diets, including nutritional and nutritious meals, staying physically active, avoiding harmful habits, and adopting wholesome daily routines.
- **Foodborne illness** caused by ingesting contaminated food containing microbes/pathogens is a further public health concern as the annual cost of treating this illness is colossal countrywide. The promotion of food safety programs and good hygiene practices effectively protects against the spread of this illness.

2.4 Threats to Public Health

Public health assures the conditions for individuals to be healthy. It requires successful countering of threats including immediate crises, e.g. pandemics, epidemics, prolonged illness, and mounting challenges, ageing, obesity, and the contaminated outcomes of a modern economy, spread via air, water, soil, or food. This section cites the major-specific threats that require the immediate attention of health organizations, medical practitioners, and social communities [10].

- **Disparities in healthcare access** are significant threats and biggest challenges globally, especially for vulnerable communities, due to various contributing factors such as cost, inadequate insurance coverage, unavailability of resources, and lack of culturally competent care. The unmet or delay in health needs leads to a substantial financial burden for individuals and countries' healthcare systems.

- **Social seclusion** and loneliness cause concern and require immediate collective actions from various health organizations and social communities. There are different serious effects of sustained social seclusion on individual mental and physical health, leading to high blood pressure, obesity, or heart diseases.
- **Violence, trauma, and sufferings** have a considerable impact on overall individual health and are increasingly essential and politically charged. Crimes such as shootings, murders, sexual assault, abuse, etc. may impact victims and individuals, and communities not directly related to or experienced the incident. Such incidents may have a lifelong impact on the health and development of various sections of society. The potential long- or short-term effects may be noticed, such as self-harm, seclusion, destructive behaviours, sleep disorders, anxiety attacks, and depression.
- **Chronic malnutrition and food uncertainty** is a significant concern worldwide. The contributing factors are low income, cost, poor urban planning, lack of transport facilities, lack of resources such as supermarkets, etc. which have enhanced the food deserts globally. The unavailability of proper nutrition and missed meals has short- and long-term impacts on our future generations' healthy development.

2.5 Global Public Health and COVID-19

The recent pandemic has accentuated the significance of capitalizing in public health infrastructure and public health systems. The demand is to ascertain possible outbreaks of such pandemics and diseases as early as possible, the complete proof systems to respond to those diseases, strategies to educate the public about programs, and policies designed to help individuals (Fig. 2.4).

The pandemic has further fueled highlighting the significant risks to global public health. The inequalities in healthcare access across the globe are a much deeper concern in light of existing pandemic. The lack of availability of testing capabilities or resources and co-morbidities in certain situations has amplified challenges for the healthcare system in the present crisis [8] (Fig. 2.5).

The social distancing to curtailing the spread of infection amplifies social seclusion, notably for elderly persons, physically and mentally challenged. The pandemic has emphasized the embracing of digital transformation with virtual check-ins, telemedicine, and teletherapy.

The pandemic has lifted the risk of increased domestic violence and food insecurity due to disrupted supply chains. The poor outcomes and impact of the current pandemic are beyond measure; it demands the most vital steps for bringing the crisis under control [11].

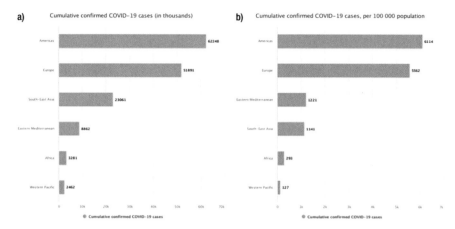

Fig. 2.4 Confirmed COVID-19 cases [1]. *Source* WHO Statistics (May 2021). https://www.who.int/publications/m/item/weekly-epidemiological-update-on-covid-19---25-may-2021

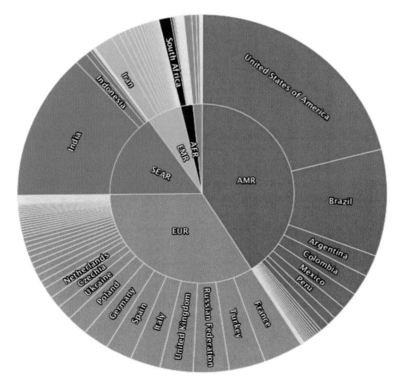

Fig. 2.5 Collective verified COVID-19 by location [1]. *Source* WHO Statistics (May 2021) https://www.who.int/publications/m/item/weekly-epidemiological-update-on-covid-19---25-may-2021

2.6   Obstacles to Practical Problem-Solving in Public Health

Public health has a reputation of triumph that should be a source of satisfaction. Still, challenges that can erode current and future public health capacities should be found and confronted regularly [3, 7]. Few identified obstacles that lead to ineffective action includes the following:

- Lack of unanimity about mission and content among various stakeholders.
- Individual decision-making, devoid of essential data, and information
- Lack of amicable relations at different levels of government.
- Lack of capacity and inability to carry out essential tasks related to public health such as assessment, policy development, and services assurance.
- Public health unawareness.
- Lack of effective and/or consistent interactions between technical scientists and the public (via states persons).

2.7   Reinforcing Preparedness for Health Emergencies and Resilience

To repair and reinforce the damage due to the COVID-19 pandemic, countries and various stakeholders need to improve their preparedness for health emergencies. Preparedness is a collective obligation across governments, the private sector, NGOs, and individuals. Emphasis should be on achieving equitable access to vaccines and treatments to weaker and vulnerable communities of society and strengthening the health system to deal with such pandemics in the future [9, 10].

Further, the use of advanced technologies such as Artificial Intelligence and data analytics may strengthen the capacity of the country's health data and information systems. Countries can efficiently cope with emergencies and alleviate the harm to the population by carefully preparing local communities, promptly responding during crises and supporting resilience.

2.8   Summary

Public health plans focus on major public health issues, e.g. depression, anxiety, drug abuse, obesity, etc. Health organizations need to be accommodating to deliver the needs of vulnerable communities, which may shift as new economic, social, or population health issues evolve.

The next chapter will focus on AI-driven solutions for open public health issues. It will discuss the influence of AI in the development of future healthcare delivery systems.

Additional Byte -💡-

According to United Nation the revocation of health services due to pandemic could lead to a 100% surge in malaria fatalities in sub-Saharan Africa.
Source https://www.weforum.org/agenda/2020/09/global-health-facts-un-sdgs/.

References

1. World health statistics 2021: monitoring health for the SDGs, sustainable development goals. World Health Organization, Geneva. 2021. Licence: CC BY-NC-SA 3.0 IGO
2. The disarray of public health: a threat to the health of the Public https://www.ncbi.nlm.nih.gov/books/NBK218222/. Accessed 20 May 2021
3. https://www.who.int/news-room/spotlight/10-global-health-issues-to-track-in-2021. Accessed 20 May 2021
4. Global health issues to track in 2021. https://www.who.int/news-room/spotlight/10-global-health-issues-to-track-in-2021. Accessed 20 May 2021
5. Global health. https://www.healthypeople.gov/2020/topics-objectives/topic/global-health. Accessed 20 May 2021
6. St Leger L (2001) Schools, health literacy and public health: possibilities and challenges. Health Promot Int 16(2):197–205. https://doi.org/10.1093/heapro/16.2.197
7. https://www.who.int/news-room/fact-sheets/detail/food-safety. Accessed 20 May 2021
8. Schneider M-J (2021) Introduction to public health. Jones & Bartlett. ISBN 9781284197594
9. Griffiths S, Hunter D, New perspectives in public health. Taylor and Francis
10. Detels R, Beaglehole R, Lansang MA, Gulliford M, Oxford textbook of public health. Oxford University Press. https://doi.org/10.1093/med/9780199218707.001.0001
11. Gaur L, Solanki A, Wamba SF, Jhanji NZ, Advanced AI techniques and applications in bioinformatics. CRC Press. ISBN: 978-0-367-64169-6 (hbk). https://doi.org/10.1201/9781003126164

Chapter 3
AI Solutions to Public Health Issues

3.1 AI in Healthcare: Need and Opportunities

Healthcare systems and providers realize intensified capacity, supply, and workforce challenges, particularly with the COVID-19 pandemic. Ensuring access to health services is the foundation of successful health response. In precarious and conflict-affected countries, acts of aggression during the COVID-19 pandemic have already withdrawn hundreds of medical services and relentlessly thwarted the comeback.

The COVID-19 pandemic has occasionally created unpleasant environments for healthcare providers who have reported instances of violence, discrimination, and harassment.

Simultaneously, digital transformation is making an exponential increase in health data. With digitization and connectivity becoming ubiquitous, collecting and analysing vast amounts of information about individual and population health is possible. AI offers unprecedented prospects to put all the gathered data into meaningful and reasonable use, which can help physicians, clinicians, healthcare workers, and patients to make more rapid, effective, and informed decisions. The potential of AI is to facilitate devices, systems, software, and services to be context-aware, precise, personalized, predictive, and pre-emptive. It is simpler to convert data into actionable insights for precision and personalized healthcare across the health continuum with proper AI application. Apart from improving the accuracy of healthcare, AI can enhance doctors' experience by being more available for patients by spending less time focusing on data and records [1].

AI can help exempt clinicians from more tedious and routine tasks and increase engagement with the patient in a more precise and personalized way, potentially increasing value over time. Rather than looking at AI as a replacement, it should be perceived as a compliment and an augmenting factor. With the augmented intelligence of AI, it is possible to make a difference in effective patient management and move towards the human-centered approach of AI.

3.2   AI Investment in Healthcare Business

The use of AI in healthcare is not a new endeavour, the Food and Drug Administration (FDA)-approved algorithms have been used since 1998 to detect cancers in medical images. With the emergence of new technologies such as cloud computing and digitalization, efforts are much simpler than before and have improved access to data and computation speed.

Investors realizing the colossal potential that AI solutions can extend for improving patient care, intensifying the reach of services and lessening healthcare costs.

According to the start-up health insights, 2020 is the most funded year in history for health technology. The pandemic has speeded up the stride of AI adoption, and healthcare advisors are confident AI can unravel specific toughest challenges, including COVID-19 tracing and vaccines. The extensive capacity of digital health applications and the prospective volume of the healthcare market are propelling substantial surge of investment in health technology. The number of contracts and overall subsidies has risen precipitously over the past decade [2, 3] (Table 3.1).

The anticipated ventures varied from digital diagnosis to clinical decision support and precision medicine. Regardless of the confidence about the potential for AI, officials across industries deem more regulations are needed and prodigiously believe the government has a crucial role to play in policing AI technology. Several healthcare officials are still too cautious in trailing with AI due to privacy and data integrity concerns. The unfortunate existence of numerous structural silos creating data sharing unfeasible [4, 5] (Fig. 3.1).

Since health AI is emerging in evolving markets, no comparable data countrywide is available, though development is anticipated in specific disciplines post-COVID-19 [6, 7].

Table 3.1 Health innovation funding in health-tech companies

Year	Total raised	Project size
2010	$1.1B	150
2011	$2.1B	282
2012	$2.3B	395
2013	$2.8B	554
2014	$7.1B	580
2015	$6.1B	498
2016	$8.2B	602
2017	$11.8B	838
2018	$14.7B	791
2019	$13.9B	719
2020	$21.0B	770

Source Start-up Health Insights, data as of 2020, URL: https://www.startuphealth.com/2020-yearend-insights-report)

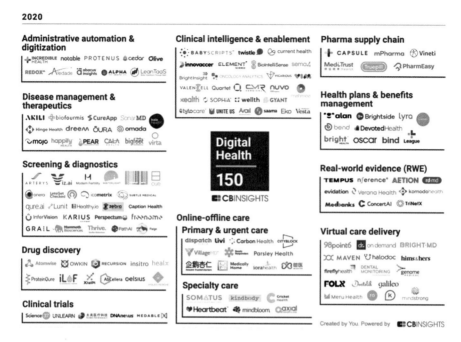

Fig. 3.1   Healthcare AI start-ups. *Source* CB Insights, 2020. "Digital Health 150: The Digital Health Startups Transforming the Future of Healthcare" https://www.cbinsights.com/research/artificial-intelligence-startups-healthcare/

3.3   AI in Healthcare: Opportunities

AI applications in healthcare varied from incorporating algorithms for analysing chest X-rays (CXR) and CT scans [8–10], detecting cancer in mammograms [11, 12], identifying brain tumours [12, 13] on magnetic resonance images (MRI), retinal imaging [14], and predicting the development of Alzheimer's disease [15] from positron emission tomography (PET). Further, applications are demonstrated in pathology spotting, cancerous skin lesions, interpreting retinal imaging, detecting arrhythmias, and identifying hyperkaliemia from electrocardiograms. Moreover, AI has assisted in tumour detection from colonoscopy, enhancing genomics analysis, identifying genetic situations from facial form, and evaluating embryo quality to augment in vitro fertilization success.

3.3.1   AI-Based Medical Imaging

AI-based medical imaging solutions are being developed on a substantial amount of medical data to automate image analysis and diagnosis. The primary division of medical imaging constitutes breast imaging, cardiovascular imaging, lung imaging, and neurological imaging. The algorithm's output may supplement the analysis made by a radiologist to drive efficiency and decrease human error.

There is also a prospect for fully automated solutions to automatically read and interpret a scan without human supervision, which could help facilitate instant interpretation in resource-constraint geographies. Latest demonstrations of improved tumour detection on MRIs and CTs exemplify the advancement towards new opportunities for cancer impediment.

AI-based solutions have aided to enhancements in the precision, economy, and welfare of patient. It has also enabled definitive diagnosis, timely treatment, efficiency in the radiology workflow, and quality control. Undoubtedly, these automated solutions will strengthen radiologists in clinical diagnosis and clinical decision support, thus reducing fault and malpractice costs.

Let us take a few medical imaging tools for multiple different projects: infectious disease (e.g. COVID-19 and TB) and diabetic retinopathy.

(a)   TB, a prominent infectious airborne bacterial disease, affects the lungs. The disease is propagated person-to-person in droplets as a TB patient sneezes, coughs, or talks. It is potentially a severe condition, but the proper treatment can cure it at the right time. Thus, the diagnosis of TB at early stages is a crucial public health challenge. Diagnosing TB at the early stage is difficult because its symptoms can mimic those of specific respiratory diseases. The conventional and cost-effective screening technique, chest X-rays, is one way to improve the screening process. However, resource-constrained countries are facing a shortage of experts for interpretation. Hence, WHO recently endorsed the usage of computer-aided detection (CAD) for screening and triaging [8–10].

(b)   The COVID-19 pandemic has created a lot of havoc globally. AI leverages the unparalleled stride of attempts to tackle the COVID-19 pandemic situation. It is efficaciously used in the identification of infected clusters, monitoring of patients, prediction of the impending outbreaks, mortality risk, resource allocation, maintenance of health records, pattern analysis, and trend analysis. Healthcare professionals use various AI-driven systems for the detection and quantification of COVID-19 cases from CXRs and CT scans [16–22].

Even though both are categorized as a pulmonary abnormalities, their clinical manifestations vary. Therefore, a generic AI tool may not be a good idea since algorithms must learn their respective expressions. Data availability is another concern that makes AI-driven tools limited to education and training—not all tools can be commercialized. Cross-population test/train models are always of importance. Researchers have been progressing by taking a concept of active learning, where AI-driven tools learn data from the beginning of the day they generated [17, 22, 23].

(c)   **Diabetic retinopathy analysis**

Early screening of diabetic retinopathy is crucial to prevent vision loss and blindness in diabetic patients. It can be an additional opportunity to detect other diseases of the eyes as well as cardiovascular diseases. The demand for such screening is growing due to the advent of digital photography and digital recording of retinal images through picture archiving and communication systems (PACS). Screening using fundus photography followed by manual image analysis requires experts and is a costly affair. The deep learning algorithms show great promising results with increased quality outcomes at less cost.

In coming years, AI-driven medical imaging will foster facilitating complex imaging of organs, soft tissues, bones, and complete body structures, and processing speed, displaying parameters like 3D/4D, faster, and accurate workflow automation [23–28].

3.3.2 AI in Drug Discovery

According to the AI Index report 2021, the AI investment in drug design and discovery increased significantly in 2020 (USD 13.8 billion), which was 4.5 times higher than the previous year [1]. Many pharma companies presently leverage AI to assist with drug discovery and enhance the prolonged timelines and practices entwined to uncovering and transporting medications to market.

AI-driven drug discovery has opted to crowdsource PostEra platform "Moonshot" to combat the COVID-19 pandemic. Over 500 international scientists join this initiative to accelerate the development of an antiviral against the COVID-19 pandemic (Fig. 3.2).

Apart from that, AI is used in distinct pharmaceutical industry sectors, including drug repurposing, enhancing pharmaceutical productivity, and clinical trials; it facilitates lowering human workload and accomplishing targets briefly.

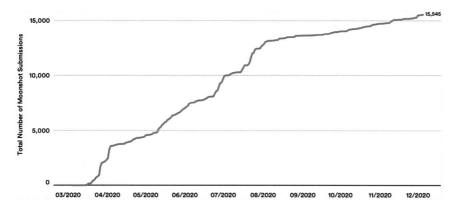

Fig. 3.2 Postera: total number of moonshot submissions. *Source* PostEra, 2020 | Chart: 2021 AI Index Report https://aiindex.stanford.edu/wp-content/uploads/2021/03/2021-AI-Index-Report_Master.pdf

The contribution of AI ranges from the development of a pharmaceutical product, rational drug design, assist in decision-making, determine the appropriate treatment for a patient, involving personalized medicines, and handle the clinical data generated and apply it for potential drug development.

AI solutions are being developed to discover new prospective therapies from massive databases of information on existing medicines, which could be revamped to target critical threats such as the Ebola virus. It can increase the efficiency and accomplishment rate of drug development, quickening the process to bring new drugs to market in response to deadly disease threats [2–4].

3.3.3 AI in Clinical Practices

It should not be encouraged and appropriate that AI-enabled diagnostics should replace human decision-making. However, AI-enabled diagnostics can help specialists, especially in resource-constrained healthcare systems such as laboratories and imaging centers.

AI solutions can provide immediate support to clinicians to help classify at-risk patients by scrutinizing historical patient data. It includes re-admission risks and underscoring patients that have arisen chance of returning to the hospital within 30 days of discharge. Several companies and health systems are developing solutions on data in the patient's electronic health record, driven partly by expanding pushback from payers on covering hospitalization costs linked with re-admission.

Although many use cases are still at early or experimental stages, AI technology can be assimilated into imaging and diagnostics processes to allow physicians and technicians to devote more time to complex cases, clinical interpretation, and patient communication [2, 3].

3.3.4 AI in Primary Care

Organizations are at work on direct-to-patient solutions to triage and give advice through chatbot interaction. It can deliver rapid, walkable access for fundamental questions and medical concerns and reduce the substantial demand of primary healthcare providers. In few cases, it provides essential assistance that otherwise is difficult for populations in remote or under-served areas. Though these technologies are promising, these solutions still need substantial independent validation to establish patient safety and efficacy.

3.3.5   AI in Cardiology

The early detection of atrial fibrillation (AF) is another application of AI in medicine to prevent AF-related stroke. Smartphone-based ECG monitoring and detection are used for the detection of atrial fibrillation. Further, AI has been used to predict the risk of cardiovascular disease, for instance, acute coronary syndrome and heart failure, better than traditional measures.

3.4   Using AI to Augment Public Health Issues

Global health leaders have realized the potential of AI-enabled tools throughout the public health crisis, especially in sharing biological information globally, research, collaboration, and various other operation pursuits.

Data suggest that the leading causes of death, such as heart diseases, cancer, respiratory diseases, and stroke, have been reduced due to aggressive education and awareness campaigns. Though the cost of these campaigns is very high, and leverage of AI can help pinpoint specific demographics or geographies where population health issues exist can help target and precisely implement education and treatment programs and reduce expenditure [28].

Using AI and ML to evaluate large datasets, health experts can discover at-risk populations for several diseases, from diabetes to heart disease. Opioid addiction is another area that can benefit from AI. Prescription and illegal opioids are the main reasons for drug overindulge deaths in the US itself. While opioid overdoses are a challenge across the country, particular counties, states, and regions suffer significantly higher rates of opioid abuse and misuse than others. AI can help identify these regions; good campaigns and education programs can be run only for those regions for better results. AI holds great potential to make population health programs more targeted to achieve future goals [15, 29].

3.5   Leveraging AI for the Future of Healthcare

With a surfeit of issues to conquer, propelled by an ageing population and growing rates of chronic diseases, the necessity for new groundbreaking solutions in healthcare is apparent.

In the coming years, the safest prospects for AI in healthcare are hybrid models, where clinicians are backed in diagnosis, treatment preparation, and ascertaining risk factors but preserve fundamental responsibility for the patient's care. It will eventually help faster adoption and deliver considerable improvements in patient outcomes and operational efficiency at magnitude (Fig. 3.3).

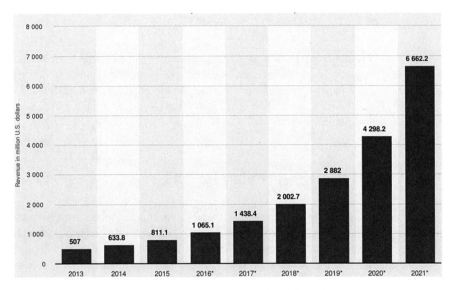

Fig. 3.3 Revenue from AI-driven system in healthcare (in Million). *Source* IP Pragmatics, Frost and Sullivan, Statistics 2019 https://www.frost.com/news/press-releases/600-m-6-billion-artificial-intelligence-systems-poised-dramatic-market-expansion-healthcare/

The potential of AI technologies in improving the speed, affordability, remote access, and preventative focus of health-tech innovations entails an ecosystem in which investors, regulators, technologists, medical and research professionals, and consumer advocates develop agreement on regulatory frameworks; as well as to administer these technologies and approve on the ethical restrictions of their applications. However, the future of healthcare and AI is profoundly interconnected.

3.6   Summary

AI-driven healthcare solutions have created a buzz for good reasons. With the availability of massive data, skilled workers, and emerging technologies, the potential of AI can be unlocked for a better future of public health. The bond of AI and healthcare seems to be profound in the coming years with technology and data growth advancements.

The next chapter uncovers the relationship between AI and sustainable public health. It will delve into making the path for a responsible, sustainable, and broad use of AI for public healthcare.

Additional Byte -♀-

What is ICD?

ICD stands for International Classification of Diseases, a global healthcare classification system, maintained by WHO for diagnosis, health management and clinical purposes. The eleventh revision of the ICD, the ICD-11, was accepted by WHO's World Health Assembly (WHA) on 25 May 2019 and will officially come into effect on 1 January 2022.
    Source "World Health Assembly Update, 25 May 2019". 25 May 2019.

References

1. Zhang D, Mishra S, Brynjolfsson E, Etchemendy J, Ganguli D, Grosz B, Lyons T, Manyika J, Carlos Niebles J, Sellitto M, Shoham Y, Clark J, Perrault R (2021) The AI index 2021 annual report. AI Index Steering Committee, Human-Centered AI Institute, Stanford University, Stanford, CA
2. Baig MA, Almuhaizea MA, Alshehri J, Bazarbashi MS, Al-Shagathrh F (2020) Urgent need for developing a framework for the governance of AI in healthcare. Stud Health Technol Inform 272:253–256. https://doi.org/10.3233/SHTI200542 PMID: 32604649
3. Gunasekeran DV, Tseng RMWW, Tham YC et al (2021) Applications of digital health for public health responses to COVID-19: a systematic scoping review of artificial intelligence, telehealth and related technologies. npj Digit Med 4:40. https://doi.org/10.1038/s41746-021-00412-9
4. Esmaeilzadeh P (2020) Use of AI-based tools for healthcare purposes: a survey study from consumers' perspectives. BMC Med Inform Decis Mak 20:170. https://doi.org/10.1186/s12911-020-01191-1
5. Mrazek M, O'Neill F. Artificial intelligence and healthcare in emerging markets. https://www.ifc.org/wps/wcm/connect/56acc8c7-28ba-40ff-96cb-80ebfdad179d/EMCompass_Note+91-Healthcare+and+AI_FIN-Sept-web.pdf?MOD=AJPERES&CVID=njAgxHj. Accessed 23 May 2021
6. Healthcare AI investment will shift to these 5 areas in the next 2 years: survey. https://www.fiercehealthcare.com/tech/healthcare-executives-want-ai-adoption-to-ramp-up-here-s-5-areas-they-plan-to-focus-future. Accessed 23 May 2021
7. Ghosh S, Bandyopadhyay A, Sahay S, Ghosh R, Kundu I, KC Santosh (2021) Colorectal histology tumor detection using ensemble deep neural network. Eng Appl Artif Intell 100:104202
8. KC Santosh, Vajda S, Antani SK, Thoma GR (2016) Edge map analysis in chest X-rays for automatic pulmonary abnormality screening. Int J Comput Assist Radiol Surg 11(9):1637–1646. https://doi.org/10.1007/s11548-016-1359-6
9. Karargyris A, Siegelman J, Tzortzis D, Jaeger S, Candemir S, Xue Z, KC Santosh, Vajda S, Antani SK, Folio LR, Thoma GR (2016) Combination of texture and shape features to detect pulmonary abnormalities in digital chest X-rays. Int J Comput Assist Radiol Surg 11(1):99–106. https://doi.org/10.1007/s11548-015-1242-x
10. KC Santosh (2020) COVID-19 prediction models and unexploited data. J Med Syst 44(9):170. https://doi.org/10.1007/s10916-020-01645-z
11. Ghosh S, Chaki A, KC Santosh (2021) Improved U-net architecture with VGG-16 for brain tumor segmentation. Phys Eng Sci Med. https://doi.org/10.1007/s13246-021-01019-w
12. Ghosh S, KC Santosh (2021) Tumor segmentation in brain MRI: U-nets versus feature pyramid network. CBMS 2021:31–36

13. KC Santosh, Ghosh S, Bose M (2021) Ret-GAN: retinal image enhancement using generative adversarial networks. CBMS 2021:79–84

14. KC Santosh, Antani SK (2018) Automated chest X-ray screening: can lung region symmetry help detect pulmonary abnormalities? IEEE Trans Med Imaging 37(5):1168–1177. https://doi.org/10.1109/TMI.2017.2775636

15. KC Santosh (2020) AI-driven tools for coronavirus outbreak: need of active learning and cross-population train/test models on multitudinal/multimodal data. J Med Syst 44(5):93. https://doi.org/10.1007/s10916-020-01562-1

16. KC Santosh, Ghosh S (2021) Covid-19 imaging tools: how big data is big? J Med Syst 45(7):71. https://doi.org/10.1007/s10916-021-01747-2

17. Das D, KC Santosh, Pal U (2020) Truncated inception net: COVID-19 outbreak screening using chest X-rays. Phys Eng Sci Med 43:915–925. https://doi.org/10.1007/s13246-020-00888-x

18. Mukherjee H, Ghosh S, KC Santosh (2021) Deep neural network to detect COVID-19: one architecture for both CT scans and chest X-rays. Appl Intell 51(5):2777–2789. https://doi.org/10.1007/s10489-020-01943-6

19. Mukherjee H, Ghosh S, KC Santosh (2021) Shallow convolutional neural network for COVID-19 outbreak screening using chest X-rays. Cogn Comput. https://doi.org/10.1007/s12559-020-09775-9

20. KC Santosh (2020) COVID-19: prediction, decision-making, and its impacts, book series in lecture notes on data engineering and communications technologies. Springer Nature. https://doi.org/10.1007/978-981-15-9682-7

21. Joshi A, Day N, KC Santosh (2020) Intelligent systems and methods to combat COVID-19. Springer briefs in applied sciences and technology. ISBN 978-981-15-6571-7 (print). 978-981-15-6572-4 (online). https://doi.org/10.1007/978-981-15-6572-4

22. Das D, KC Santosh, Pal U (2020) Cross-population train/test deep learning model: abnormality screening in chest X-rays. CBMS 2020:514–519

23. Ruikar DD, KC Santosh, Hegadi RS, Rupnar L, Choudhary VA (2021) 5K+ CT images on fractured limbs: a dataset for medical imaging research. J Med Syst 45(4):51

24. Ruikar DD, KC Santosh, Hegadi RS (2019) Automated fractured bone segmentation and labeling from CT images. J Med Syst 43(3):60:1–60:13

25. Ruikar DD, Hegadi RS, KC Santosh (2018) A systematic review on orthopedic simulators for psycho-motor skill and surgical procedure training. J Med Syst 42(9):168:1–168:21

26. Ruikar DD, Sawat DD, KC Santosh, Hegadi RS (2018) 3D imaging in biomedical applications: a systematic review. J Med Imaging Artif Intell Image Recogn Mach Learn Tech

27. Ruikar DD, KC Santosh, Hegadi RS (2018) Segmentation and analysis of CT images for bone fracture detection and labelling. Med Imaging 130–154

28. Gaur L, Singh G, Agarwal V (2021) Leveraging artificial intelligence tools to combat the COVID-19 crisis. In: Singh PK, Veselov G, Vyatkin V, Pljonkin A, Dodero JM, Kumar Y (eds) Futuristic trends in network and communication technologies. FTNCT 2020. Communications in computer and information science, vol 1395. Springer, Singapore. https://doi.org/10.1007/978-981-16-1480-4_28

29. Gaur L, Bhatia U, Jhanjhi NZ et al (2021) Medical image-based detection of COVID-19 using deep convolution neural networks. Multimed Syst. https://doi.org/10.1007/s00530-021-00794-6

Chapter 4
AI in Sustainable Public Healthcare

4.1 Background

AI is precipitously starting a new edge in sustainable public health. As the AI revolution transforms the healthcare sector, it could signify a perfect future where humanity co-exists harmoniously with machines or herald a dystopian world filled with dispute, impoverishment, and suffering if not used responsibly [1].

AI-driven applications in poor resource settings are still at a nascent stage. In 2017, the UN convened a global meet to discuss the advancement and prospects of AI applications to optimize public health services, reduce poverty, and provide a wide variety of vital public services. The broader suitability of AI in public health is due to various factors such as ubiquitous, appropriateness, flexibility, learning from more comprehensive datasets, and past patterns. It can imitate the cognitive function of human minds as well. Fast learning from vast datasets can help health experts discover at-risk populations for chronic diseases and decrease the financial burden. Compared to traditional mechanisms, AI algorithms can help detect threats and suggest suitable interventions based on past data to prevent disasters and create a healthy future for the public [2].

4.2 AI for Resolving Global Public Health Challenges

Sustainable Development Goal (SDGs) number 3 aims to "ensure healthy lives and target No. 3.3 reads", ending the scourges of AIDS, TB with "End TB Strategy", malaria and overlooked tropical diseases and prevent hepatitis, water-borne diseases, and other infectious diseases [1, 3] (Fig. 4.1).

According to the global TB report 2020, the Countries with the highest TB burden (at least 100 000 incident cases) are India, Indonesia, China, the Philippines, Pakistan,

K. Santosh and L. Gaur, *Artificial Intelligence and Machine Learning in Public Healthcare*, SpringerBriefs in Computational Intelligence, https://doi.org/10.1007/978-981-16-6768-8_4

33

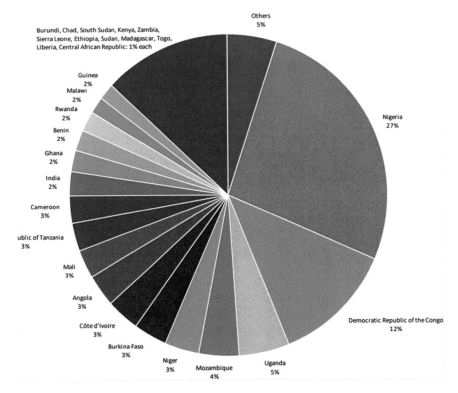

Fig. 4.1 Global distribution of malaria cases, by country, 2019. *Source* World Health Statistics 2021 https://www.who.int/data/gho/publications/world-health-statistics

Nigeria, Bangladesh, and South Africa. The health scale in SDGs has been significantly widened compared to the Millennium Development Goals (MDGs), now encompassing non-communicable diseases, the well-being of the elderly, mental health, substance abuse, tobacco smoking, environmental health hazards, injuries, and road traffic accidents [4] (Fig. 4.2).

WHO and the international community have co-operatively established global policies towards attaining the global health-related targets exemplified within the SDGs and the WHO Triple Billion targets? These strategies concentrate on halting several contagious diseases by 2030, e.g. TB, HIV, malaria, NTDs, and polio, emphasizing continued investments in nations [5] (Table 4.1).

SDG goal three heavily advocates capitalizing on human health to boost economic growth, safeguard the environment, and decrease poverty. The investment in public health goals such as vaccination, safe water can bring higher than their costs. Besides, unsustainable manufacturing, expenditure, and environmental pollution have a long-term effect on public health. Thus, sustainable public health is a need of an hour [6–8].

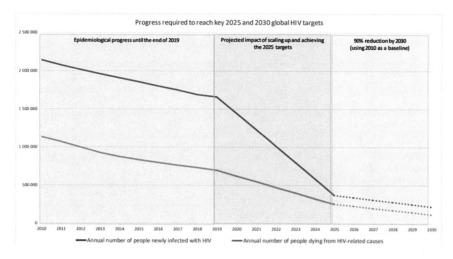

Fig. 4.2   Global trends (HIV incidence and mortality) and progress expected to attain key 2025 and 2030 global targets, 2010–2030. *Source* World Health Statistics 2021 https://www.who.int/data/gho/publications/world-health-statistics

AI holds great promise to achieve sustainable public health. The diligent use of AI can have an advantage for development practitioners and beneficiaries.

- AI and big data technologies demonstrated colossal potential in the early detection of epidemics by tracing online queries on disease symptoms using social media platforms [9].
- The initial warning and detection of biosecurity threats and epidemics of influenza may be possible by investigating online queries.
- TB is one of the leading causes of death worldwide. The use of deep learning techniques for early detection and diagnosis is becoming prevalent among the researcher's community. The advances in AI technology can help reduce these curable diseases and help achieve public health targets. For example, medical imaging tools can be considered [10–13].
- Robust and responsive AI-enabled platforms can connect to various patient databases and analyze data, such as blood pathology, genomics, radiology images, and medical history, to discover hidden patterns [14, 15].
- AI is used for the identification and classification of patterns for conjunctivitis.
- The child-growth monitor uses AI algorithms to discover malnutrition dependably. The processing of such data and algorithm locally on the smartphone in resource constraints countries will be advantageous. It will also protect the privacy of patients.
- AI-based wearable device Orcam (a tiny television camera attached to the frame of eyeglasses for optical character recognition (OCR) by a microchip) converts the text, patterns, images into words heard through an earphone for artificial vision. It is providing encouraging results for blind patients.

Table 4.1 Global efforts and strategies to eradicate/eliminate major communicable diseases by 2030

	Milestones	2030 Goal	2030 SDG target
End TB strategy (8)			
TB deaths	2020: ↓ 35% 2025: ↓ 75%	↓ 95%	"End the epidemic of TB across all countries"
TB incidence rate	2020: ↓ 20% 2025: ↓ 50%	↓ 80%	
TB-affected families facing catastrophic costs due to TB (%)	2020: 0% 2025: 0%	0%	
Global health sector strategy on HIV 2016–2021 (9)			
New HIV infections	2020: <500 000/year	↓ 90%	"End the epidemic of HIV across all countries"
AIDS-related deaths	2020: <500 000/year	↓ 90%	
Global AIDS strategy 2021–2026 (10)			
New HIV infections	2025: <370 000/year	↓ 90%	"End the epidemic of HIV across all countries"
AIDS-related deaths	2025: <250 000/year	↓ 90%	
Global technical strategy for malaria 2016–2030 (11)			
Malaria incidence	2020: ↓ 40% (at least) 2025: ↓ 75% (at least)	↓ 90% (at least)	"End the malaria epidemic across all countries"
Malaria deaths	2020: ↓ 40% (at least) 2025: ↓ 75% (at least)	↓ 90% (at least)	
Countries eliminating malaria	2020: 10 countries 2025: 20 countries	35 countries	
Road map for neglected tropical diseases (NTDs) 2021–2030 (12)			
People requiring interventions against NTDs	Disease-specific targets set for each NTD include 2023 and 2025 milestones	↓ 90%	"End the NTDs epidemics across all countries"
Disability-adjusted life years related to NTDs		↓ 75%	
Countries eliminating al least one neglected tropical disease		100	
NTDs eradicsted		2	
Polio endgame strategy 2019–2023 (13)			
Wild poliovirus transmission	2030: Eradication of polio		

Source World Health Statistics 2021 https://www.who.int/data/gho/publications/world-health-statistics

- Another AI application is digital surgery robots. These AI-driven robots have provided the prospect of telemedicine and remote surgery for simple procedures.
- AI can lead from the forefront for diagnostics and the interpretation of pathology results and image classification. It would help clinicians available to provide continuing guidance to patients. Hence, AI can fill disparities in information, identify patterns and connections, and help predict risks and prospects and ultimately increase diagnosis and treatment efficacy.
- Mobile health using a smartphone is widely acceptable in low-income countries and rural areas. The AI-driven healthcare Chatbots, virtual avatars, and characters can tremendously help populations suffer from stigmatizing pathologies, reduce accessibility issues, and provide initial assessment and recommendations about medication and tests. It can significantly save time and enables healthcare practitioners to spend quality time with patients.
- AI-enabled mobile apps and wearables could enable healthy decision-making by supervising behaviours and amassing personal data such as mental health and social networks. Community health workers can use it to improve the provision of health services within resource-poor settings.
- AI automated translations solutions can significantly reduce language barriers and improve the accessibility of services in remote areas globally.

4.3 Challenges

There are a plethora of factors implicated in establishing sustainable health systems:

- AI data-driven techniques are exceptionally prepared to confront challenges, such as long queues, fear of unreasonable bills, the long-drawn and excessively intricate appointment process, not getting access to the right healthcare specialist. The consumer's viewpoint is one of the major contributing factors in establishing sustainable health. Consumers are responsible for a more significant share of total healthcare costs worldwide. It is imperative to provide value to them for better sustainability.
- The development of expert systems supporting clinical decision-making is a vital challenge; the major hindrance is the precise definition of clinical problems for proper implementation.
- The non-availability of vast and quality datasets is another major challenge for the broader generalization of results. The ML algorithms need massive datasets for the identification of risk factors or the diagnosis of diseases. Additionally, a better diagnosis does not warrant access to suitable treatment alternatives. While remote diagnostics and ML applications might help detect diseases, therapeutic services may or may not be implemented.
- Another major challenge is the broader adaptability of clinical NLP systems to varied healthcare settings. The hand-penned local linguistic health records also create a significant challenge in the diagnosis of the diseases. However, WHO has

encouraged the embracing of regulated medical terminologies or regional data dictionaries to handle these issues.

- Lack of proper infrastructure in developing countries may lead to fragile communication networks, cause problems in electronic health records, and deliver primary healthcare services.
- The electronic health records are available in various portals, and ingesting data and recognizing patterns from these incongruent sources creates uncertainty which is challenging to achieve with standard statistical modelling techniques. Thus, AI solutions are required for solving such high-scale problems [14, 15].
- Other challenges are associated with data sharing, ethical issues, and privacy of vulnerable populations suffering from stigmatized pathologies. The robust principles and policies should be the priority for government and policymakers. The responsible use and privacy standards must be strictly followed to protect the population from hackers, structural violence, and various other threats and eventually bring the question of human rights to security.
- There is a possibility of over-reliance on AI that may lead to a destruction of clinical skills, critical thinking skills, and community health practices [6–8, 14, 15].

4.4   Summary

The AI tools and techniques in sustainable public health healthcare are still in their formative years. Despite the shortcomings, they are advantageous in providing comprehensive information on individuals' health and predicting population health risks. Its utilization for medicine alongside public health is likely to increase significantly. Simultaneously, it is also essential to maintain confidentiality, security, ownership of patient data. It is worth declaring that techniques that enable AI models to learn from datasets without conceding their privacy are becoming progressively more critical shortly.

Effective implementation requires an understanding of the local, social, epidemiological, and political contexts. Thus, the responsible and ethical use of AI in public health will help attain the health-related goals in SDG and achieve sustainable public health.

The potential of AI is not limited to detection and modelling; instead, it can also potentially predict future patients' likelihood of having diseases provided early screening or regular annual examination. Furthermore, they may be able to model "why" and in "what circumstances" conditions are expected to happen and, thereby, can help guide and prepare both doctors to intervene (in a personalized manner) even before an individual begins exhibiting symptoms.

Furthermore, there is an urgent need to develop a more comprehensive, all-inclusive, consumer-centered approach that concentrates on wellness, prevention, and continuous health management across different sectors. The "New Model" of health should also involve economic, social, and other facets of individuals' lives.

The next chapter will focus on the role of AI in precision medicine and explore the integration of precision medicine into healthcare for accurate diagnoses, predicting the probability of diseases before symptoms appear.

Additional Byte -$\bigcirc$-

Human-caused emissions of carbon dioxide need to fall 45% from 2010 levels by 2030 and reach net-zero around 2050 to limit climate change catastrophe. If people worldwide switched to energy efficient light bulbs the world would save 105 billion euros annually.
Source https://sumas.ch/sustainability-facts/.

References

1. World health statistics (2021) Monitoring health for the SDGs, sustainable development goals. World Health Organization, Geneva 2021. Licence: CC BY-NC-SA 3.0 IGO https://www.who. int/data/gho/publications/world-health-statistics
2. Alami H, Rivard L, Lehoux P et al (2020) Artificial intelligence in health care: laying the Foundation for Responsible, sustainable, and inclusive innovation in low- and middle-income countries. Global Health 16:52. https://doi.org/10.1186/s12992-020-00584-1
3. Goralski MA, Tan TK (2020) Artificial intelligence and sustainable development. Int J Manage Educ 18(1):100330. ISSN 1472–8117. https://doi.org/10.1016/j.ijme.2019.100330.
4. Benke K, Benke G (2018) Artificial intelligence and big data in public health. Int J Environ Res Public Health 15:2796. https://doi.org/10.3390/ijerph15122796
5. Seke K, Petrovic N, Jeremic V et al (2013) Sustainable development and public health: rating European countries. BMC Public Health 13:77. https://doi.org/10.1186/1471-2458-13-77
6. Artificial Intelligence, Public Trust, and Public Health https://blogs.cdc.gov/genomics/2020/ 09/17/artificial-intelligence/. Accessed on May 26, 2021
7. Stefan Buttigieg MD (2021) Rising to the challenge: better public health with Artificial Intelligence. https://blog.infermedica.com/rising-to-the-challenge-better-public-health-with-artificial-intelligence-part-1/. Accessed on 26 May 2021
8. Schmidt H, Gostin LO, Emanuel EJ (2015) Public health, universal health coverage, and Sustainable Development Goals: can they co-exist? 386(9996): P928–930. https://doi.org/10. 1016/S0140-6736(15)60244-6
9. Gaur L, Singh G, Agarwal V (2021) Leveraging artificial intelligence tools to combat the COVID-19 crisis. In: Singh PK, Veselov G, Vyatkin V, Pljonkin A, Dodero JM, Kumar Y (eds) Futuristic trends in network and communication technologies. FTNCT 2020. Communications in Computer and Information Science, vol 1395. Springer, Singapore. https://doi.org/10.1007/ 978-981-16-1480-4_28
10. KC Santosh, Antani SK (2018) Automated chest X-ray screening: can lung region symmetry help detect pulmonary abnormalities? IEEE Trans Med Imaging 37(5): 1168–1177. https://doi. org/10.1109/TMI.2017.2775636
11. KC Santosh, Vajda S, Antani SK, Thoma GR (2016) Edge map analysis in chest X-rays for automatic pulmonary abnormality screening. Int J Comput Assist Radiol Surg 11(9):1637–1646. https://doi.org/10.1007/s11548-016-1359-6
12. Karargyris A, Siegelman J, Tzortzis D, Jaeger S, Candemir S, Xue Z, KC Santosh, Vajda S, Antani SK, Folio LE, Thoma GR (2016) Combination of texture and shape features to detect pulmonary abnormalities in digital chest X-rays. Int J Comput Assist Radiol Surg 11(1):99–106. https://doi.org/10.1007/s11548-015-1242-x

13. Gaur L, Bhatia U, Jhanjhi NZ et al (2021) medical image-based detection of COVID-19 using deep convolution neural networks. Multimedia Syst. https://doi.org/10.1007/s00530-021-007 94-6
14. Gaur L, Solanki A, Wamba SF, Jhanjhi NZ (2021) Advanced AI techniques and applications in bioinformatics. CRC Press. ISBN: 978-0-367-64169-6. https://doi.org/10.1201/978100312 6164
15. Kaswan KS, Gaur L, Dhatterwal JS, Kumar R (2021) AI-based natural language processing for the generation of meaningful information electronic health record (EHR) data. In: Advanced AI techniques and applications in bioinformatics. CRC Press. ISBN: 978–0–367–64169–6. https://doi.org/10.1201/9781003126164

Chapter 5
AI in Precision Medicine

5.1 Background

The field of medicine is expanding towards prevention, personalization, and precision. AI is a vital means to attain contemporary medicine.

Precision medicine is a massive development in healthcare caused by expertise acquired from sequencing the human genome. It is advanced to understand how the juncture of panomics data blended with patients' medical history, social factors, and environmental understanding specifically depicts health, disease, and therapeutic alternatives for affected persons [1].

Precision medicine will enable healthcare providers to realize and offer information that substantiates the medical decision based on individual traits. The advancements in new data analytics techniques have helped in achieving personalized care. The primary technologies involved in the development of medicine are genomics, biotechnology, artificial intelligence. For instance, the merging of soaring-output genotyping and electronic health records provided researchers with an exceptional prospect to derive additional phenotypes from clinical and biomarker data. In combination with electronic health records, these phenotypes may authenticate the need for different therapies or remedies to enhance diagnoses of disease modifications (Fig. 5.1).

The efficacy of treatments and diagnosis of evidence-based medicine is done through alternative therapies such as modern medicines. For instance, patients with hypersensitive effects after consuming cough syrups are not recommended cough syrups, and a somewhat alternative solution is provided. They used AI algorithms that use disruptive technologies like cheap genome sequencing, advanced biotechnology, health sensors for the patients, electronic health records, hand-held medical devices, etc., for data collection and suggestions based on individual characteristics.

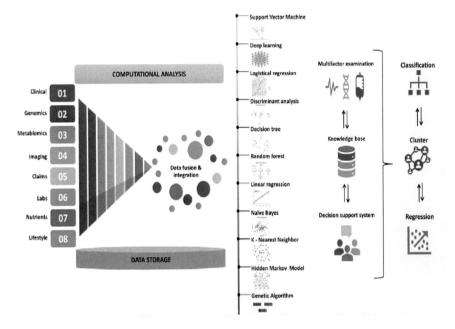

Fig. 5.1 AI algorithms for precision medicine [2]

5.2 Precision Medicine and AI

The main aim of precision medicine is to predict the finest and safest treatment for the individual. The next-generation sequencing (NGS) technology has revolutionized medical research and facilitated multi-layer experiments that assimilate genomic data, such as DNA sequence, RNA sequence, and multi-omics data (e.g. proteome, epigenome, and microbiome). The drug reactions blend with genomic, epigenomic, transcriptomic, proteomic, metabolomic profiling data to present accurate predictions to the distress. The ML algorithms can be exploited in modelling to predict genomic characteristics for practice and drug response prediction.

With precision medicine and the development of next-generation sequencing (NGS), genomic reports of individuals are now exploited for risk prediction, disease diagnosis, and the development of personalized medication and remedies. The application of ML in gene expression (for genomic profiles) is not a brand-new idea. Traditionally, it was done with microarrays and now with RNA sequence.

Traditionally, the genomic sequencing analysis was done by experts, and curation endeavours rely on protein structure, functional studies that predict the practical impact of genetic alteration; however, the progression of AI technologies impacts the field. For AI to significantly impact precision medicine requires significant computing power and powerful self-learning deep learning algorithms that use physicians' cognitive capabilities. The AI algorithms helped physicians in diagnoses in

Table 5.1 List of companies using a form of AI to improve healthcare and medicine

Company	The main area of research
Google DeepMind	Mining medical records
Verily	Wearable sensors
IBM Watson	Mining medical records
Careskore	Quality of care
Zephyr Health	Identifying therapies
Sentrian	Remote patient intelligence platform
3Scan	Radiology
Enlitic	Radiology
Arterys	Radiology
Atomwise	Drug development
Deep Genomics	Genomics

Source Mesko [7]

cardiology, dermatology, and oncology, and it is imperative to use these algorithms under the guidance of physicians.

Precision medicine requires various disruptive technologies such as AI and data analytics to stimulate building cures, perform treatment, and provide care. For instance, in cancer genomics, variant classification, clinical relevance, literature validation, and summarization are conventionally performed by healthcare experts. AI technologics can be utilized as a support expert to validate the diagnosis. AI solutions should support the proficiencies of physicians and are not intended to reinstate the conventional physician–patient relationship [3] (Table 5.1).

5.3 Critical Success Factors of AI for Precision Medicine

With the evolution of technologies, the performance of AI algorithms will improve in times to come. The two leading factors that can enhance AI algorithms' performance are vast amounts of data and relevance. Big data is imperative for AI algorithms to perform optimally. Undeniably, much of the recent attempt in precision medicine is fixated on acquiring bigger sample sizes, extensive DNA sequence data, electronic health records, and mobile health records (Fig. 5.2).

The accurate data is essential to augment the predictability of the model substantially. Consequently, the erroneous data can considerably influence the model's integrity and even establish biases [4].

Relevancy of data is another very critical factor to the disease of concern from disease-applicable tissues. Recent AI algorithms relied heavily on DNA sequence data, where most common conditions are broadly considered to stem from both genetic and environmental aspects and their connections.

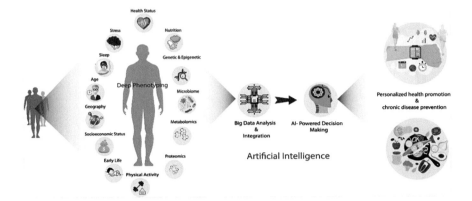

Fig. 5.2 AI and chronic disease prevention [9]

Disease-causing environmental and lifestyle factors are tough to measure. Thus, helpful genomics is an apt substitute because they quantify aggregate impacts of environmental factors on the genome and provide biological links between DNA sequences, ecological factors, and the disease. The valuable genomic records can take the types of epigenetic mutations of the DNA, profiles of RNAs (mRNA, microRNA, lncRNA, etc.), proteins, and small metabolites, and physiological function. This functional genomic is very popular in precision medicine of cancer. The studies now utilize functional genomics to apprise precision medicine apart from cancerous diseases such as kidney disease [5].

5.4 Growing Role of Disruptive Technologies in Precision Medicine

With the emergence and involvement of big giants such as Google (DeepMind Project) and IBM (Watson for oncologists and medical sieve) in AI research, the panic and question started to ponder among clinicians and other healthcare experts about their existing field. For Instance, Medical Sieve is competent to support clinical decision-making in radiology and cardiology. The "cognitive health assistant" can investigate radiology images to identify and uncover troubles more rapidly and reliably.

Deep Genomics intends to detect patterns in vast datasets of genetic evidence and medical archives, exploring mutations and ties to disease for precision medicine.

However, precision medicine requires numerous disruptive technologies to develop treatments, practice medicine, and deliver care. Though data analysis techniques are now very sophisticated, physicians' skill support is essential and cannot be superseded [6].

5.5 Challenges to AI Adoption in Healthcare

With Industry 4.0, the era of AI is evident nowadays. AI can assist throughout the medical gamut from investigation to diagnosis, therapy, and post-cancer medication. Undoubtedly, AI is driving the transformation in healthcare towards precision medicine, and digital health has become crucial for providing best practices in healthcare. The various unprecedented challenges need to be tackled before diving blindly into the pool of algorithms.

With the advancements in AI technologies, ethical, legal, privacy, and security also comes. AI is yet not a complete proof system and has severe shortcomings in healthcare. A few but the majority of us have the following concerns:

- Development of full proof mechanism to check false predictions made by AI algorithms.
- Development of secure data protection algorithms and reliable sharing while respecting citizens privacy issues.

There is an urgent need for international standardization and regulations. Thus, these unprecedented challenges posed by digital health should be addressed to ensure AI safety and favourable influence on healthcare [7].

5.6 Ethical Issues

There are pressing apprehensions about the usage of AI in precision medicine, such as bias and prejudice values which AI algorithms may learn and overfitting issues leading to unfair or inaccurate predictions. There is a possibility that a specific patient population is not included in the training set and leads to bias. The study predicted the probability of death for pneumonia patients to ascertain whether the patient was conceded into the hospital or treated as an outpatient mistakenly indicated to treat asthma patients as outpatients. The error occurs due to inadequate representation in the dataset. Similarly, prejudiced values can occur. AI can learn pre-existing disparities from a society characterized in the training set, resulting in a bias towards traditionally underprivileged populations. In addition, data can be swayed and misconstrued. These issues can be resolved by introducing high ethical standards to mitigate bias when AI is used for precision medicine. The policymakers and government are putting efforts to address AI's potential social, moral, and economic impacts and working towards developing a "good AI society" to release the enormous advantages of AI, including progress in big data-based precision medicine [8].

5.7   Future Synergies Between AI and Precision Medicine

Disruptive technologies like genomics, biotechnology, wearable sensors, or AI have significantly impacted precision medicine. They are gradually leading to personalized medication and point-of-care and creating multi-omics data for analytics [9, 10].

- Genome-apprised suggesting was among the most primitive examples of the conjunction between AI and precision medicine, with proven effective and high-throughput genome analysis.
- Radio genomics is a new precision medicine exploration field, concentrates on instituting connections between cancer imaging features and gene expression to envisage a patient's risk of developing toxicity following radiotherapy. Understanding the reaction to therapy can help clinicians selecting the right treatment strategy.
- Incorporating environmental considerations in therapy planning is an added advantage in precision medicine such as homelessness in some patients, transportation, providing medication that requires refrigeration and availability of electricity, and availability of expertise in remote locations. AI has provided several instances of boosting diagnostic competencies in resource-poor settings, which may transform into superior patient classification and additional personalized therapy planning.
- Clinical factors are essential to effective therapy planning, such as age, co-morbidities, organ function, and genomic and social aspects. AI has appeared as crucial support in the classification of patients for therapy.
- Computerized speech analytics may provide statistics for assessing and discovering early dementia, minimal cognitive deficiency, Parkinson's disease, and other mental ailments.

Thus, the synergy between AI and precision medicine has enormous potential. Its influence on the healthcare system supports the decisive goal of preventing and early detection of diseases and reducing cost and the disease burden for the public.

5.8   Summary

With the digitalization of health, disruptive technologies have begun to make sophisticated methods accessible to medical specialists and their patients. These technologies, such as genomics, biotechnology, wearable sensors, AI, have created the foundation of precision medicine.

The next chapter will emphasize the societal impact of AI on public health. The AI technology is criticized for being prejudice, less confidential, less secrecy, low explainability, low interpretability. The chapter will elaborate and concentrate on societal problems concerning AI application in healthcare.

Additional Byte-

Based on the findings of a genetic test, some medicines may be recommended that can prolong the life of a cancer patient by months or even years.

Currently, the cost to sequence an entire human genome is $5,000. The expected cost may be reduced to $1,000 in coming years.

Source https://magazine.wharton.upenn.edu/digital/facts-and-fears-about-personalized-medicine/.

References

1. Mesko B (2017) The role of artificial intelligence in precision medicine. Expert Rev Precis Med Drug Dev 2(5):239–241. https://doi.org/10.1080/23808993.2017.1380516
2. Williams AM, Liu Y, Regner KR, Jotterand F, Liu P, Liang M Artificial intelligence, physiological genomics, and precision medicine. https://doi.org/10.1152/physiolgenomics.00119.2017
3. Johnson KB, Wei W-Q, Weeraratne D, Frisse ME, Misulis K, Rhee K, Zhao J, Snowdon JL Precision medicine, AI, and the future of personalized health care. https://doi.org/10.1111/cts.12884
4. Filipp FV (2019) Opportunities for artificial intelligence in advancing precision medicine. Curr Genet Med Rep 7:208–213. https://doi.org/10.1007/s40142-019-00177-4
5. Bhinder B, Gilvary C, Madhukar NS (2021) Elemento O Artificial intelligence in cancer research and precision medicine. https://doi.org/10.1158/2159-8290.CD-21-0090. Published April 2021
6. Uddin M, Wang Y, Woodbury-Smith M (2019) Artificial intelligence for precision medicine in neurodevelopmental disorders. npj Digit Med 2:112. https://doi.org/10.1038/s41746-019-0191-0
7. Mesko B (2017) The role of artificial intelligence in precision medicine. Exp Rev Precis Med Drug Dev. https://doi.org/10.1080/23808993.2017.1380516
8. Santus E, Marino N, Cirillo D, Chersoni E, Montagud A, Santuccione Chadha A, Valencia A, Hughes K, Lindvall C (2021) Artificial intelligence–aided precision medicine for COVID-19: strategic areas of research and development. J Med Internet Res 23(3):e22453. https://doi.org/10.2196/22453,PMID: 33560998; PMCID: 7958975
9. Subramanian M, Wojtusciszyn A, Favre L et al (2020) Precision medicine in the era of artificial intelligence: implications in chronic disease management. J Transl Med 18, 472 (2020). https://doi.org/10.1186/s12967-020-02658-5
10. Gaur L, Solanki A, Wamba SF, Jhanjhi NZ Advanced AI techniques and applications in bioinformatics. CRC Press. ISBN: 978-0-367-64169-6 (hbk). https://doi.org/10.1201/9781003126164

Chapter 6
Societal Impact:- AI in Public Health Issues

6.1 Background

AI has permeated every facet of society, fueling all from online advertisements, financial trading systems, social media apps, autonomous cars, hospitality, and now the much propaganda is around technology's algorithms corresponding the Expertise of human specialists at numerous tasks and providing a powerful signal of its impending arrival and long-term survival.

According to estimates by WHO, there is a worldwide scarcity of practitioners and the medical doctor soon, a challenge that presents a more significant danger in evolving countries. The studies demonstrated that AI has enormous potential to reduce the burden in public healthcare systems and improve patient care.

Undoubtedly, AI-driven public health research provides ground-breaking diagnostics, drug discovery, precision medicine, healthcare worker productivity, and chronic disease management. AI is grabbing significant interest from federal agencies, media and draw from society. AI can be a foremost vigour for societal good; currently, there is a substantial focus on the upcoming ethical, safety, and legal issues related to AI applications [1, 2, 2].

AI techniques are poised to perform a significant role in our society across distinct spheres involving public health. Therefore, they need to be devised to safeguard rational gains for all (Table 6.1).

6.2 AI for Social Goodness

AI is by now heroic in many fields. It can do the calculation, play chess, transliterate speech, read lips, recollect things for longer, and certainly faster and sharper than human beings. The social good uses AI cases ranging from diagnosing cancer,

Table 6.1 Benefits and perils of AI in healthcare

Benefits	Perils
Improving efficiencies for the operational management of healthcare business	The fast pace of technology and impact on decision-making
Accuracy of diagnosis and treatment in personal medicine	Privacy and security issues
Increased insights to enhance cohort treatment	Lack of regulation and bias

Source https://www2.deloitte.com/us/en/insights/industry/health-care/artificial-intelligence-in-health-care.html

pinpointing victims of online sexual abuse, catastrophe aid efforts to help sightless people navigate their surroundings.

According to the report of McKinsey, AI has vast potential throughout a variety of social domains such as education, infrastructure, environment, healthcare, data substantiation and validity, equality and inclusion, public and social and safety sector, crisis response, plus economic empowerment.

AI in public health is vital for doctors, patients, health organizations, countries at large. Public health scientists and experts have initiated employing AI for diverse tasks such as searching cyberspace for burgeoning epidemics, forecasting suicide tapping electronic health records [6, 7], and spotting threats. Intrinsically, there has been mounting positivity concerning the prospective for AI to enhance social well-being [2–4] (Table 6.2).

The famous illustrations are IBM Watson's power to identify remedies for cancer patients. Another illustration is Google Cloud's Healthcare application to collect, store, and access data with no effort. Synching up to the progress of remote alliance and care in public health, there is an upsurge in adopting AI tools, such as digital Chatbots, that help the public comprehend their symptoms and self-triage. Additionally, on-demand care is forming a vast mandate for virtual care tools through web and mobile apps. The upcoming goals to remote patient observing for consumers in the home are embedded analytics and in-home observing.

An eminent application Verily fostered by Google focuses on anticipating both noncontagious and hereditary genetic ailments. These apps empower health experts to foresee potential threats and take preventive measures before it occurs.

AI can automate healthcare administrative tasks, such as pre-approving insurance, follow-ups on unpaid bills, and storing records, to reduce healthcare professionals' workload and save cost. In addition, wearables such as Fitbit's and smartwatches use AI to monitor individual's health and send alerts to healthcare professionals about potential health issues and risks. These technologies help reduce unnecessary visits to hospitals and costs and eases the workload on healthcare professionals.

AI technology is up-and-coming for specific crises such as natural disasters and outbreaks of diseases. For example, the AI algorithm can help firefighters and saviours forecast the movement of wildfires using satellite data and help find lost people in wilds areas. In addition, computer-vision abilities have prospective

Table 6.2 AI applications for digital disruption of health

Main area	Prospective annual value by the year 2026	Main reasons for embracing
Robot aided operation	$40B	Technical innovations in robotics
Simulated nursing personal assistant	$20B	The high burden due to medical labour shortage
Organizational system	$18B	Increased portability and integration with existing infrastructure
Fraud exposure	$17B	The rise in cyber frauds and its identification mechanism
Dosage error reduction	$16B	Frequency of medical inaccuracies, which leads to substantial forfeits
Linked devices	$14B	The rise of attached devices
Clinical test participation	$13B	Patent cliff, availability of lots of data, outcome-guided method
Primary diagnosis	$5B	Data design to augment precision
Automated image diagnosis	$3B	More confidence in AI technology
Cybersecurity	$2B	Rise in infringements; pressure to protect health data

Source https://www.accenture.com/us-en/insight-artificial-intelligence-healthcare%C2%A0

usage for social good, such as recognition of people, face detection, and emotion identification appropriate in crisis response, security, equality, and education.

NLP is beneficial when data is written, like case reports, health data, newspaper sections, and messages. In addition, AI tools, principally utilizing emotion and face detection, can improve educational prospects for children with autism by providing signs to assist children in recognizing and eventually understanding family and friends' facial manifestations [2, 3, 6, 7].

6.3   Societal Concerns of AI in Public Health

Though AI has many positive potentials, there are various perils of using AI and has possible risks. It has raised concerns about the core of essential human rights safeguards such as privacy and freedom of expression. There are many instances where AI-driven, poorly designed systems can misdiagnose the diseases. The software is also criticized for being culturally biased in few cases. One severe and sensational claim against the use of AI technology is that as AI increases to the point that it transcends human talents, it may come to take command over our assets and outcompete, heading to human annihilation [2, 3, 6, 7].

There are severe apprehensions concerning AI's effects on privacy, interpretability, and security.

- **Legislation**: Any AI application in healthcare practice is compelled to debate its legal restrictions and connotations. AI advancements in healthcare have remained ignorant to legal concerns, although their increased usage impacts society and is likely to knock a bit of legal fence. One extensively debated use case of AI is autonomous vehicles. Though AI algorithms are utilized to deliver automatic decision-making, and, thus, it spots these tools in legal interest. Therefore, it is advisable that healthcare experts and practitioners need to poise in AI-driven technologies' efficacy and their observance of current legislation.
- **Interpretability and explainability**: In recent times, AI-driven systems' interpretability and explainability have come to the forefront of healthcare research. The main reason is created by DL techniques (a subfield of ML). Interpretability issue is considered as a human–computer interaction challenge. The desire is to ensure that the model's outcomes can be explained to human beings despite being complex. The issue of explainability has severe concerns in medicine and has clear implications. The black box decisions by AI-based decision-making systems without coherent explanation may not promise the system's trustworthiness and may create a problematic situation for healthcare experts. Integrating expert knowledge into an AI-driven system framework may be a potential solution for improved machine–human interaction.
- **Privacy and confidentiality**: Data privacy has been the source of foremost concern for all businesses worldwide; however, healthcare is highly vulnerable to data infringements. The advancements in technology increased adoption of telecommunication, and overuse of the Internet and social networks have raised data privacy issues. It has become a critical issue in healthcare with the increased adoption of electronic healthcare data for medical practices with varying levels of security at distinct junctures. Several worldwide standards safeguard such as HIPAA and ISO, ensure the meticulous conservation and concealment of privacy and security of affected individual records. Although few researchers proposed techniques to protect a patient's data privacy and security, the research in this field is yet growing every day.

- **Ethics and Impartiality**: To make a mistake is human, yet be grateful to AI; human beings are not only to blame. Who is responsible for an accident by a self-driving car? What if an AI-driven, armed military drone attacks an enemy in miscalculation? Likewise, healthcare has to deal with similar moral questions. The core challenge is that the whole structure of healthcare is staged to achieve profit instead of raising health. The issue does not alter with the supplement of AI, but it offers a soaring prospect of getting much worse in times to come.
- **Equality/inequality**: AI has transformed the comfort with which individuals from all over the globe can retrieve information, credit, and various advances of modern-day global society and has helped in the enormous reduction of world-wide disparity and extreme scarcity. For illustration, permitting agriculturalists to realize reasonable rates, good quality yields, and access to precise meteorological conditions forecasts remotely is one positive aspect of this technology. Concurrently, there is anxiety that economic disparity could develop even further and take away the ability of one social-economic class to gain from technology [4, 5].

6.4 Challenges

The potential bottlenecks that could limit AI benefits to society are (Table 6.3).

Table 6.3 Critical barriers

Critical barriers related to Data	Data accessibility Data quality Data volume Data labelling Data availability Data Integration
Critical barriers related to Expertise	AI—expertise availability (High) AI—expertise accessibility issue AI—practitioner talent availability AI—practitioner talent accessibility
Critical barriers relation to computation	Access to technology Access to computing capacity Access to software library and other tools
Critical barriers due to organizational capability	Administrative implementation efficiency Scale AI deployment Organizational repetitiveness
Other potential barriers	Regulatory constraints Privacy concerns "Last mile" implementation challenge

Source McKinsey Global Institute Analysis https://www.mckinsey.com/featured-insights/artificial-intelligence/applying-artificial-intelligence-for-social-good

6.5 Summary

Research demonstrated the prospective advantages of AI for advancing public health. However, numerous impediments persist, and consequences ought to be clearly illustrated. Specialists emphasized the possibility for AI to enhance infection reconnaissance and health support involvements for more exploration and assessing investigations.

AI is getting hype as well as facing criticism from various stakeholders. In brief, if AI technology will unite humankind with the machine, strengthening human intelligence with artificial intelligence, the stakeholders and policymakers need to manage the risk!

Additional Byte

Therapeutic robots and the socially assistive robots help enhance the quality of life for old aged and physically confronted. Cy-borgs have been advised to accompany lonesome elderly for daily chores.

Source Tai M. C. (2020). The impact of artificial intelligence on human society and bioethics. Tzu chi medical jour-nal, 32(4), 339–343 https://doi.org/10.4103/tcmj.tcmj_71_20

References

1. Gao S, He L, Chen Y, Li D, Lai K (2020) Public perception of artificial intelligence in medical care: content analysis of social media. J Med Internet Res 22(7):e16649. https://doi.org/10.2196/16649PMID.32673231PMCID: 7385634
2. Tomašev N, Cornebise J, Hutter F et al (2020) AI for social good: unlocking the opportunity for positive impact. Nat Commun 11:2468. https://doi.org/10.1038/s41467-020-15871-z
3. GÃ³mez-GonzÃ¡lez, E., Artificial Intelligence in Medicine and Healthcare: applications, availability and societal impact, Gomez Gutierrez, E. editor(s), EUR 30197 EN, Publications Office of the European Union, Luxembourg, 2020, ISBN 978–92–76–18454–6, https://doi.org/10.2760/047666, JRC120214
4. Tomašev N, Cornebise J, Hutter F et al (2020) AI for social good: unlocking the opportunity for positive impact. Nat Commun 11(2468). https://doi.org/10.1038/s41467-020-15871-z
5. Morgenstern JD, Rosella LC, Daley MJ et al (2021) AI's gonna have an impact on everything in society, so it has to have an impact on public health: a fundamental qualitative descriptive study of the implications of artificial intelligence for public health. BMC Public Health 21:40. https://doi.org/10.1186/s12889-020-10030-x
6. Vellido A (2019) Societal issues concerning the application of artificial intelligence in medicine. Kidney Dis 5:11–17. https://doi.org/10.1159/000492428
7. AI is not a silver bullet, but it could help tackle some of the world's most challenging social problems. By Michael Chui, Martin Harrysson, James Manyika, Roger Roberts, Rita Chung, Pieter Nel, and Ashley van Heteren https://www.mckinsey.com/featured-insights/artificial-intelligence/applying-artificial-intelligence-for-social-good. Accessed 14 June 2021

Chapter 7
Case Studies—AI for Infectious Disease

7.1 Prelude

Infectious diseases are instigated by infective microbes, for instance, bacteria, viruses, worms, or fungi. The ailments can be indicative or symptomless. Specific contagious and fatal diseases like Human Immunodeficiency Virus (HIV) can be reasonably symptomless, leading to catastrophic results. These microbes may spread quickly and lead to pandemics. The subsequent disease may lead to minor to acute fatal indications.

The 1918 flu was one of the fatal of all influenza pandemics, which happened during world war I. The key reason for the dispersed was poor cleanliness and unusual troop movement. Apart from influenza, there is persistent danger from various infectious diseases such as TB, cholera, smallpox, such as severe acute respiratory syndrome, middle east respiratory syndrome, Ebola, and Zika viruses.

As infectious diseases may lead to a pandemic, the best preventive strategy is to detect potential pandemics and prevent the spread by quarantine. By barring disseminate, there is a prospect to reduce the virus's mutation and combat the virus. The best and effective means to reduce the dispersion of infection is by improving hygiene conditions and broader dissemination of vaccine campaigns. While *quarantine* is efficient in limiting the disperse of diseases, there is no efficient cure yet for various infectious diseases. The latest SARS is an exemplar of an emerging contagious illness, an extreme variation of Coronavirus scattered among continents within weeks. The multiplicative extent of the pathogen and the dispersed-out ratio of the disease are distinct among geographies pondering the disparity in the population density, demographics, ecosystems, and conduct.

As per the latest eruptions of numerous infections, risen population intensity and agility play a critical part in the spree of emergent infectious diseases, potentially leading to pandemics [1–5].

7.2   Dimensions of AI for Combating Infectious Diseases

AI is at the edge of transforming the healthcare system by concentrating; disease-focused evaluation and mediations to stimulate swifter, consistent, and cost-effective healthcare solutions for individuals' welfare at large. AI algorithms are analyzing massive data from numerous platforms of infectious diseases such as countrywide surveillance systems, genome records, epidemic enquiry reports, vaccine reports, social media platforms, net search inquiries, and vaccine statements to find the underlying developments [3, 6, 7] (Fig. 7.1).

AI is additionally facilitating in epidemic modelling and simulation of the disease spread knowledge for the policymakers to take valuable healthcare actions [8–10]. The main dimensions where AI helps fight against infectious diseases are:

- **Diagnosis**: AI is beneficial in diagnosing vast amounts of data, including image analysis such as X-rays and CT scans and may help clinicians and health experts diagnose various infectious diseases. AI and ML-driven image detection algorithms have hastened diagnosis and triage patient care to detect COVID-19 symptoms using lung images. Thus, the practitioners and healthcare experts can make quick decisions in resource-constrained areas [11–18].
- **Identification of social factors**: AI can help understand the social aspects of any new disease and its influence, diffusion, and recovery. A pandemic can be minimized by understanding individuals' demographics, lifestyle, movement patterns, and behavioural aspects. Thus, using AI-driven algorithms, it is easier and quicker to understand this vast population-related data into actionable knowledge to augment treatment programs.
- **Drug discovery**: Vaccine creation and commercialization takes years and involves a more complex inside understanding of virus genes. AI has been promising in developing models that simulate the evolution, transmission, and spread pattern of viruses and help identify the finest contenders for prospective vaccines.
- **Relief**: AI has potential in predicting the effective virus suppression and relief strategies for a particular region, such as the deployment of imaging systems to monitor social distance; thermal cameras with facial recognition to monitor

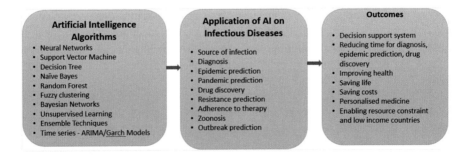

Fig. 7.1 Relation of AI algorithms and outcomes

employees' health; and traffic analysis that monitors the probable dispersion among individuals.

7.3   Case 1: AI for COVID-19 (SARS-CoV-2) Pandemic

The year 2020 has intensely transformed the way we live our natural life and carry out our daily activities. The COVID-19pandemic is a foremost worldwide challenge to public health alongside terrible social, economic, and political effects. The world has viewed numerous disease epidemics that attacked humans in the past. Even today, the organizations such as WHO and several other national authorities across the globe are struggling against these pandemics. The COVID-19 verified in the Wuhan district of China in December 2019 created havoc and continues to increase worldwide. The clinical seriousness, quick diffusion, and fatality due to COVID-19 have led the WHO to pronounce it a pandemic.

The pandemic has led to severe anxieties about healthcare systems' inability to handle the extraordinary challenge for health services, incredibly resource-constrained countries. Thus, the urgent need for tools technologies is felt across the globe to speed up diagnostic processes, augment monitoring and tracking capacities, prediction (citation, see below) detect early stages of the infection, and influence society and imitate the outcomes of a suppression policy. In addition, early detection of the disease is vital for individuals and healthcare experts to ensure sufficient patient seclusion and disease suppression [12–16].

The pandemic has accelerated the embracing of AI in various disciplines. AI technologies, anticipating offering effective and affordable simulations to tackle health and social concerns, and have indeed attracted critically affected provinces. AI-driven solutions encapsulate patients' data that enables healthcare experts to provide judgments and outline a customized treatment schedule. Primarily, the application of AI helps to find the effects of disease treatments and disease deterrence.

- **Datasets (for prediction—long-term and short-term)**
  One of the biggest challenges for the successful implementation of AI tools is the readiness of superior-quality data. Though various universities and organizations created free online resources such as:

  – Harvard Dataverse (https://dataverse.harvard.edu).
  – WorldPop (https://www.worldpop.org).

  John Hopkin Centre created the 2019 Novel Coronavirus Visual Dashboard dataset for delivering evidence instantaneously. For COVID-19, predictive modelling uses SEIR/SIR, agent-based, curve-fitting techniques/models broadly. Predictions aim at making states and citizens aware of possible threats/consequences. However, state-of-the-art prediction models are failed to exploit crucial and unprecedented uncertainties/factors, such as (a) hospital settings/capacity; (b) test capacity/rate (daily); (c) demographics; (d) population density; (e) vulnerable people; and (f) income versus commodities (poverty). Predictions can be short-term and long-term. No statistical models in the literature can make long-term predictions. The primary reason behind this is the presence of unprecedented factors [16–19].

- **AI for diagnosis of COVID-19**
  Research has proved to effectively categorize the intensity of seriousness of the illness by using CXR and CT scans image datasets and clinical blood samples. Various DL algorithms, such as CNN, Naive Bayes, SVM, RF and decision trees, are utilized to diagnose COVID-19 [12–19]. Many researchers have implemented these algorithms on different datasets to classify and predict various diseases like pneumonia. The maximum likelihood algorithms have demonstrated better results in the past for other infectious diseases. The composite of maximum likelihood AI-driven strategy worked best for SARS-COVID-19 to address the concern that arises from the small sample size, quality of data, and missing information to confirm a rapid retort to public health demands [19–22] (Fig. 7.2).

- **AI for contact tracing** is the process of locating individuals already exposed and infected with the COVID-19 virus to lessen the dispersion. The severely infected countries use digital contact tracing techniques such as mobile apps and various technologies such as Bluetooth, GPS, social graph, contact details, mobile tracking data, and card transaction data for real time and faster tracing. Furthermore, the data collected by digital apps are further analyzed using AI technologies for tracing vulnerable individuals in the contact chain.
- **AI for predicting infection AI technologies can** predict the probability of getting the COVID-19 infection. It is also possible to predict and forecast the transmission rate and improvements worldwide. The deep learning technique, such as LSTM with feedback connections, is a valuable technique to categorize, analyze, and forecast. Another method, NLP, assists predictions by congregating data connected to the deterrence and spreading of the virus in the region news report.
- **AI for drug design**: AI tools and docking applications demonstrated active results in the reusability of existing drugs for COVID-19 medication, thus helps in reducing the cost and risk involved in the development of medicine. However, the challenge associated is the availability of resources of comprehensive amalgam data and realistic implementation of the application [23].
- **AI in disease forecasting and dissemination pattern**: AI tools also help forecast the dissemination pattern of the COVID-19 virus and its spread among districts, states, and countries. AI-driven systems assist in tackling the disease spread and can be proactive in forecasting a disease outbreak.

7.4   Case 2: AI for Tuberculosis Detection

The WHO (2020) report reiterated TB, an extremely infectious disease, is among the prominent causes of fatality worldwide. In 2020 united nations' sustainable development goals (UNSDGs) and WHO's End TB policy were endorsed. Early and precise

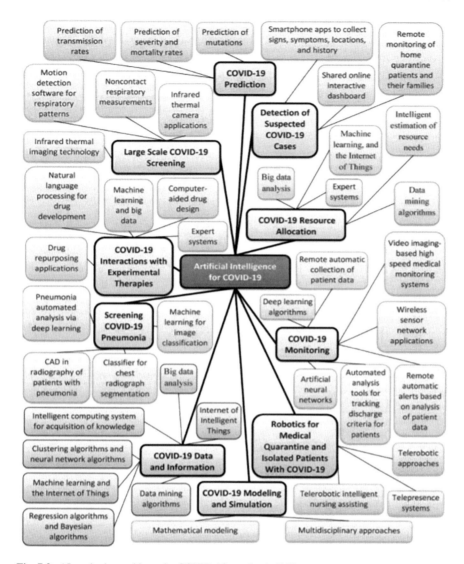

Fig. 7.2   AI methods to address the COVID-19 pandemic [11]

TB detection is crucial to accomplish control of the disease worldwide. Thus, the exploration in the medical imaging of TB has demonstrated exponential progress recently. Medical imaging is the prevalent method for examining TB; it reveals distinct patterns in the lung. The CXR and CT scans are majorly applied imaging modalities for analyzing and diagnosing pulmonary TB and are primarily used for detecting lung abnormalities [12–18]

Numerous diseases appear with similar radiologic patterns; disparity in the diagnosis of diseases ought to be contemplated while reading a CXR, involving various forms of pneumonia, occupational lung diseases, neoplastic disease, pleural effusion, and cardiac disease. The challenge confronted by different emerging nations is the shortage of competent radiologists to interpret CXR reports and CT scans. Simultaneously amid expert radiologists, the possibility of variability cannot be denied due to fatigue, perceptual biases, and cognitive biases, which may lead to errors.

Computer vision has demonstrated substantial improvement and encouraging findings isolating medical imaging features. Conventional techniques used manual feature descriptors tweaked for specific datasets. Additionally, they are trained for inconsistencies in size, positioning, and position. However, DL averted these constraints of conventional techniques across extensive feature extraction and classification.

DL-assisted detection systems for TB are comprehensively exploited by researchers and mentioned as an up-and-coming solution for clinicians' challenges in high burdened and resource-constrained countries. These techniques intend to augment clinical decision-making, assisting clinicians in administrating and focusing on high-risk cases and lowering the likelihood of misdiagnosis and suggesting additional diagnostic tests without delay. Furthermore, the prevalent algorithms of deep learning, for instance, CNN, are deemed precise, cost-effective, and necessitate minimal human mediation.However, the number of computer-aided device systems with DL technology for TB detection has increased significantly [9, 11–16].

WHO has recently advocated CAD systems for TB detection, guided by execution research and operational experiments to augment impact. In future, the correlation of demographics, clinical data, and AI abnormal scores should be explored to achieve individualized risk scores, thereby optimizing the performance of CAD systems [6, 19–23].

7.5   Case 3: AI for Influenza

Influenza is a severe respiratory contagion triggered by the influenza virus, which poses a considerable threat to public health and causes fatality each year worldwide. Influenza viruses are categorized into A, B, C, and D. Typically, seasonal flu is triggered by type A or B. H1N1 influenza is one of the nastiest flu infections. Consequently, surveillance and early detection of influenza supported by well-timed response are vital for the readiness of the influenza pandemic.

Conventionally, in epidemiology, influenza prediction is performed via diffusion system models. The traditional system faced a challenge of a time lag of approx. 1–2 weeks in publishing influenza-like illness (ILI) report and delay in optimal decision-making. Thus, attempts are made for real-time assessment of influenza activity in the preceding decade.

Google launched Google Flu to monitor the trends and predict the ILI. Subsequently, data from multiple sources such as the web, influenza surveillance data, Twitter, Wikipedia, and electronic health records were unified with scientific models to trace illness activities for better and accurate predictive outcomes.

A range of AI algorithms has recently been harnessed to influenza-like illness guesstimate, encompassing the autoregressive integrated moving average (ARIMA), Lasso regression, Support Vector Machine (SVM), AdaBoost, and deep learning techniques. Though, few methods were able to forecast seasonal influenza patterns and the unusual variants effectively. Furthermore, a small number of studies have centered on enhancing influenza projection accuracy using multiple data sources [10, 23].

7.6 Summary

AI-driven systems are a crucial and essential technology that transformed the healthcare sector for global advantage. AI applications are vast and are pivotal in addressing infectious diseases such as TB, Influenza, and COVID-19. Apart from the advancement of biological research, the AI applications compliment the quicker analysis of infectious diseases' vast data to offer speedier decision-making capabilities to support the policymakers, medical professionals, and healthcare institutions for retorting any impending conditions.

The next chapter will focus on the significant issues related to AI. The chapter will elaborate on the various concerns related to privacy, security, and ethical dimensions. It will also deliberate on the solutions and recommend ways for resolving them.

Additional Byte

Universal health coverage (UHC) implies that all entities and populations obtain the health services they want without enduring financial hardship. It comprises the complete continuum of important, quality health benefits, from health promotion to prevention, medication, rehabilitation, and relaxing care across the life path.

Source https://www.who.int/news-room/fact-sheets/detail/universal-health-cov erage-(uhc).

References

1. Mei X, Lee HC, Diao Ky et al (2020) Artificial intelligence-enabled rapid diagnosis of patients with COVID-19. Nat Med 26:1224–1228. https://doi.org/10.1038/s41591-020-0931-3
2. Lalmuanawma S, Hussain J, Chhakchhuak L (2020) Applications of machine learning and artificial intelligence for Covid-19 (SARS-CoV-2) pandemic: a review. Chaos, Solitons Fractals 139:110059. https://doi.org/10.1016/j.chaos.2020.110059
3. Malik YS, Sircar S, Bhat S, Ansari MI, Pande T, Kumar P, Mathapati B, Balasubramanian G, Kaushik R, Natesan S, Ezzikouri S, El Zowalaty ME, Dhama K (2020) How artificial intelligence may help the Covid-19 pandemic: pitfalls and lessons for the future—reviews in medical virology. Adv Online Publ e2205. https://doi.org/10.1002/rmv.2205

4. Gaur L, Singh G, Agarwal V (2021) Leveraging artificial intelligence tools to combat the COVID-19 Crisis. In: Singh PK, Veselov G, Vyatkin V, Pljonkin A, Dodero JM, Kumar Y (eds) Futuristic Trends in Network and Communication Technologies. FTNCT 2020. Communications in Computer and Information Science, vol 1395. Springer, Singapore. https://doi.org/10.1007/978-981-16-1480-4_28

5. Piccialli F, di Cola V, Giampaolo F et al (2021) The role of artificial intelligence in fighting the COVID-19 pandemic. Inf Syst Front. https://doi.org/10.1007/s10796-021-10131-x

6. Gaur L, Bhatia U, Jhanjhi NZ et al (2021) Medical image-based detection of COVID-19 using deep convolution neural networks Multimedia Syst. https://doi.org/10.1007/s00530-021-007 94-6

7. Mottaqi MS, Mohammadipanah F, Sajedi H (2021) Contribution of machine learning approaches in response to SARS-CoV-2 infection. Inform Med Unlocked 23:100526. ISSN 2352-9148. https://doi.org/10.1016/j.imu.2021.100526

8. Liu C, Zhou Q, Li Y, Garner LV, Watkins SP, Carter LJ, Smoot J, Gregg AC, Daniels AD, Jervey S, Albaiu D (2020) ACS Cent Sci 6(3):315–331. https://doi.org/10.1021/acscentsci.0c0 0272

9. Zeng D, Cao Z, Neill DB (2021) Artificial intelligence-enabled public health surveillance—from local detection to global epidemic monitoring and control. Artif Intell Med 437–453. https://doi.org/10.1016/B978-0-12-821259-2.00022-3

10. Agrebi S, Larbi A (2020) Use of artificial intelligence in infectious diseases. Artif Intell Prec Health 415–438. https://doi.org/10.1016/B978-0-12-817133-2.00018-5

11. Jain K (2020) Artificial intelligence applications in handling infectious diseases. Prim Health Care 10(5):351

12. KC Santosh (2020) AI-driven tools for coronavirus outbreak: need of active learning and cross-population train/test models on multitudinal/multimodal data. J Med Syst 44(5):93. https://doi.org/10.1007/s10916-020-01562-1

13. KC Santosh, Ghosh S (2021) Covid-19 imaging tools: how big data is big? J Med Syst 45(7):71. https://doi.org/10.1007/s10916-021-01747-2

14. Das D, KC Santosh, Pal U (2020) Truncated inception net: COVID-19 outbreak screening using chest X-rays. Phys Eng Sci Med 43:915–925. https://doi.org/10.1007/s13246-020-008 88-x

15. Mukherjee H, Ghosh S, KC Santosh (2021) Deep neural network to detect COVID-19: one architecture for both CT scans and chest X-rays. Appl Intell 51(5):2777–2789. https://doi.org/10.1007/s10489-020-01943-6

16. Mukherjee H, Ghosh S, KC Santosh (2021) Shallow convolutional neural network for COVID-19 outbreak screening using chest X-rays. Cogn Comput. https://doi.org/10.1007/s12559-020-09775-9

17. KC Santosh (2020) COVID-19: prediction, decision-making, and its impacts, book series in lecture notes on data engineering and communications technologies. Springer Nature. https://doi.org/10.1007/978-981-15-9682-7

18. Joshi A, Day N, KC Santosh (2020) Intelligent systems and methods to combat COVID-19, Springer briefs in applied sciences and technology. ISBN: 978-981-15-6571-7 (print), 978-981-15-6572-4 (online). https://doi.org/10.1007/978-981-15-6572-4

19. KC Santosh (2020) COVID-19 prediction models and unexploited data. J Med Syst 44(9):170. https://doi.org/10.1007/s10916-020-01645-z

20. KC Santosh , Sameer K (2018) Antani: automated chest X-ray screening: can lung region symmetry help detect pulmonary abnormalities? IEEE Trans Med Imag 37(5):1168–1177 (2018). https://doi.org/10.1109/TMI.2017.2775636

21. KC Santosh , Vajda S, Antani SK, Thoma GR (2016) Edge map analysis in chest X-rays for automatic pulmonary abnormality screening. Int J Comput Assist Radiol Surg 11(9):1637–1646 (2016). https://doi.org/10.1007/s11548-016-1359-6

22. Karargyris A, Siegelman J, Tzortzis D, Jaeger S, Candemir S, Xue Z, KC Santosh , Vajda S, Antani SK, Folio LR, Thoma GR (2016) Combination of texture and shape features to detect pulmonary abnormalities in digital chest X-rays. Int J Comput Assist Radiol Surg 11(1): 99–106 (2016). https://doi.org/10.1007/s11548-015-1242-x
23. Gaur L, Solanki A, Wamba SF, Jhanjhi NZ. Advanced AI techniques and applications in bioinformatics. CRC Press, ISBN: 978-0-367-64169-6 (hbk). https://doi.org/10.1201/978100 3126164

Chapter 8
Privacy, Security, and Ethical Issues

8.1 Background

AI has spread its wings rapidly in healthcare, from automating drudgery and regular medical procedures to supervising patients and medical reserves. The potential benefits of AI in medicine are pressing the limits of human performance, democratizing medical expertise and merit, regulating the regular tasks, managing medical resources, and adopting revenue amplifying systems. While developers create AI systems to take on these tasks, numerous consequences and challenges arise, comprising the danger of injuries to patients from AI system oversights, the threat to patient secrecy of data procurement and AI interpretation, etc. The potential and well-known risks are biases and inequality, errors, privacy concerns, less availability of data and danger of replacing human expertise, etc. Balance out the perils and incentives of AI in healthcare will require a collaborative effort from technology developers, regulators, end-users, consumers.

8.2 Data Privacy and Protection Issues

Experts have raised apprehensions about the privacy consequences of healthcare data storage and data security systems, and AI is foremost in that discussion.

The biggest shortcoming of AI algorithms is the need for the volume of datasets collected in clinical trials for better diagnosis and generalization. In a few medical fields, e.g. obstetrics, ophthalmology is at the forefront of AI-driven systems due to the overall accessibility of massive, well-curated imaging datasets. The ready availability of anonymized datasets is always a boon for technological advancement. However, it also represents a significant risk of compromising patient privacy regarding their social security, financial status, etc.

K. Santosh and L. Gaur, *Artificial Intelligence and Machine Learning in Public Healthcare*, SpringerBriefs in Computational Intelligence, https://doi.org/10.1007/978-981-16-6768-8_8

Elimination of all possibly distinguishable data from large datasets can be an intimidating task. It will always persist a speculative threat of re-identification. Even in ophthalmology, it is currently feasible to employ facial identification software for 3D restorations of CT of the head. The aspects from the periocular section have been employed to detect the stage of patients using ML algorithms. The demographics, e.g. gender, age, and cardiovascular danger factors, have been discovered from fundus snapshots. It is not limited to medical images; rather, it may be feasible to distinguish entities by association with other datasets, which usually accrues over time (Fig. 8.1).

The current laws cannot protect individual health. Even a study of the University of Berkeley stated that developments of AI had delivered the Health Insurance Portability and Accountability Act of 1996 (HIPAA) antiquated. The healthcare data holds incredible value for AI companies, and compromising privacy and ethical norms are not very shocking; the recent pandemic has also aggravated the challenge.

Healthcare companies, insurance organizations, biopharma firms, and stakeholders store consumer data beyond demographics, preferences, or likes/dislikes.

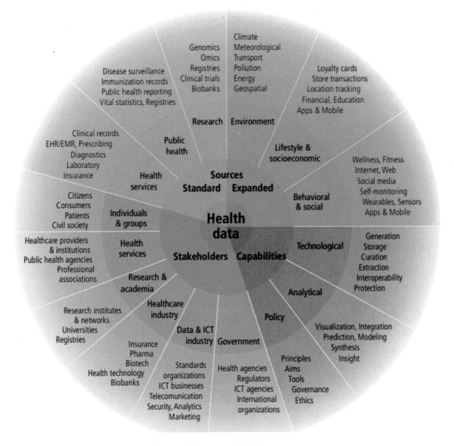

Fig. 8.1 Heath data ecosystem. *Source* Vayena et al. [1]

It contains patient's data on symptoms, medications, and different health matters. The HIPAA healthcare privacy regulations are unable to cover these technology companies. It merely safeguards patient health data from organizations that provide healthcare services, e.g. insurance companies and hospitals.

Let us take a famous case of Facebook "suicide detection algorithm" in 2017 to promote suicide awareness and protection, which used an AI algorithm to gather individual posts (without consent) and check their mental state and probability to commit suicide. AI in healthcare focuses on analyzing consumer health data to improve outcomes by suggesting diagnoses, reading medical device images, accelerating medical research and development, and more. Shockingly, this algorithm does not come under the jurisdiction of HIPPA.

HIPAA regulations even do not apply to genetics testing companies, e.g. Ancestry and 23andMe. As any rules and regulations do not bind these companies, they may sell the customer data to pharmaceutical and biotechnology firms. The information stored with these big companies is susceptible and may reveal a plethora of information about an individual ancestry, risk of diseases, e.g. celiac, Alzheimer's and Parkinson's, etc. Though, on the one hand, it seems to have a positive impact. However, insurance companies may take advantage of this information, subject to selection bias, and charge higher premiums [1].

8.3 Security Issues

AI in healthcare demonstrates potential, but security anxieties prevail [2]. Few examples are highlighted just to portray the maturity level of AI technology:

- Google Home, Alexa, Siri are extensively used by consumers nowadays. These applications use AI and ML algorithms extensively as part of its applications. These AI algorithms are limited to talking about weather forecasts or setting reminders, or playing music. They are far better at performing complex and cognitive tasks beyond the capability of a human being.
- The automotive industry has leveraged AI to present driverless cars.
- Healthcare bot is a new emerging paradigm in the healthcare sector, is an AI application for better interaction through chat windows and websites. It helps in providing appointments, follow-up appointments. No doubt, these use cases enhance customer service; offer 24/7 support for essential requirements, e.g. scheduling, billing, and clinical demands; and lessen the global administrative expenditures for hospitals.
- Wearables (e.g. Fitbit's, smartwatches, etc.), are nowadays personal life coaches, which several hospitals have pioneered as a part of their general care. However, with today's strong AI abilities and mobile apps, the affected role can advise several data elements seized on their cell phone or wearable appliances. It may be related to treatment adherence or a message that fosters fitness pursuits and healthy

patterns. The customized experience for each patient by healthcare providers offers pre-emptive warnings that can be transmitted in return to physicians.

- The advanced analytics of AI is used in oncology to help discover deformities in X-rays and MRIs in genomics to execute complicated processing and precision medicine to produce highly tailored treatments for patients. For instance, IBM Watson, the AI, has successfully applied its ability to practice structured and unstructured patient data to deliver testimony-based medication commendations for cancer patients.

Even with these promising indications and encouraging uses of AI in healthcare, the considerable risk of security persists, making healthcare professionals anxious about AI getting into the domain of patient care. The following section highlights the security challenges that ought to be surmounted before physicians will embrace the technology.

- There is an urgent need to protect patient health data under federal law and substantial financial and legal penalties for any breaches and failure to maintain its integrity. The necessity of one regulation across the access of numerous health datasets includes data stored in the vendor's data centres. The data stored on vendor's data centres are the primary security concern and the potential threat of data breaching.
- Another area of concern is the absence of interoperability among AI vendors. Hospitals throughout the globe confront the task of not being able to efficiently exchange patient health data across other healthcare organizations, despite the accessibility of data standards throughout the world. Companies like IBM or Microsoft provide health-linked customer services utilizing AI; the prospect of these organizations sharing data is very thin due to competition and proprietary technology. It can be handled by putting policies that necessitate these platforms to assemble current interoperability obligations and precisely facilitate data interchange.
- The reliability of algorithms and computers are always in question for decades, and many recent incidents have fueled it further. These malfunctions can lead to catastrophic penalties if AI recommends the incorrect medication or provides a patient with the wrong diagnosis. Nevertheless, AI could ultimately push to a phase where it can be reliable once it has demonstrated its safety and inclination for patient care with fewer errors than human experts.
- AI technology may mimic human behaviour and interact naturally with humans. The emotional responses expressed in voice tones or text have been engineered based on human emotional reactions. However, it can never replace the several judgments that physicians make based on their gut feeling and intuitions. Numerous well-known scientists and admired public figures such as Stephen Hawking, Bill Gates, and Elon Musk have said that AI could grow to be so persuasive and self-aware that it may put its pursuits ahead of humans [2].

8.4   Ethical Dimensions of AI

The application of AI in healthcare has colossal potential to transmute it for the better, but it also enhances the following ethical challenges:

- AI ethics lacks benchmarks and consensus that can measure or assess the relationship between broader societal discussions about technology development and the development of the technology itself. The applications (e.g. imaging, diagnostics, and robot surgery) may alter the patient–expert connection. The question of concern is, "how will the use of AI to support the care of patients boundary with the values of informed consent?" To what extent does a clinician need to disclose that they cannot fully interpret the diagnosis/treatment recommendations by the AI? How much transparency is required?
- The excessive use of an app such as Chatbots and health apps raise questions for bioethicists about user agreements and their relationship to informed consent. Do consumers satisfactorily comprehend that the impending use of the AI health app or Chatbot may be conditional on accepting changes to the terms of service? How tightly should user contracts be like notified consent records? What would an ethically responsible user agreement resemble in this context?
- Safety and transparency are primary ethical concerns. To appreciate the potential of AI, the developers need to focus on two essential aspects: the reliability and validity of the datasets and their transparency. Transparency creates trust among patients and healthcare specialists, which is vital for the success of AI in healthcare (Fig. 8.2).
- The AI is also criticized for a risk for biases and prejudice. Any AI algorithm can only be as reliable, efficient, and reasonable as its trained data. Many examples have confirmed that algorithms can demonstrate biases that can ensue in inequality

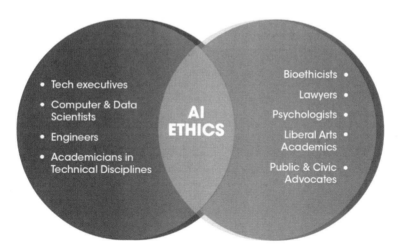

Fig. 8.2   AI ethics and disparate stakeholders [10]

concerning ethnic backgrounds and skin colour or gender. Biases can also occur concerning other characteristics such as age or disabilities. The justifications for such prejudices vary and may be complicated. They may result from the datasets themselves, from how data experts select and analyze the data, from the perspective in which the AI is used, etc. Therefore, AI developers must be mindful of this risk and curtail potential prejudices at each phase in product development. In cases of "black box" algorithms, many researchers have claimed that explainability is essential when an AI makes health suggestions, particularly identifying biases.

- The data breach incident happened in July 2017, where personal data of circa 1.6 million patients was provided to Google DeepMind by the UK Information Commissioner's Office (ICO) without consent. It is a famous case of data sharing and AI. It is fundamentally imperative to provide accurate information to the patients to foster trust between technology and the system [3].

Ethical principles for applying AI for health and added domains are anticipated to steer developers, clients, and regulators in developing and administering the design and operation of such technologies. These principles also aim to accentuate matters that occur from using a technology that could amend relations of ethical connotation [4] (Fig. 8.3).

Consequently, the principles are significant for all investors who pursue a direction in the accountable development, deployment, and assessment of AI technologies for health, comprising clinicians, systems developers, health scheme administrators, policymakers in health agencies, and governments. These should inspire and support governments and public sector societies to keep speed with the rapid development of AI technologies through regulation encourage medical specialists to use AI technologies aptly [5].

Fig. 8.3 Healthcare data transparency

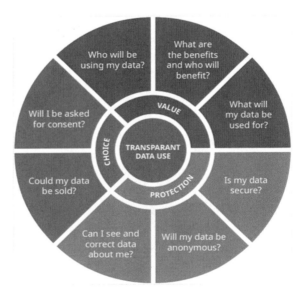

While ethical principles are widespread, their enactment may diverge to cultural, religious, and social environments [6].

- Protect autonomy principle requires that any extension of machine autonomy not undermine human independence. It implies that humans should persist in complete control of healthcare systems and medical judgments in healthcare. AI skills should not be utilized to investigate or exploit humans in a healthcare system without legitimate enlightened sanction.
- These technologies should not harm individuals. They should comply with regulatory constraints for security, precision, and effectiveness before deployment, and procedures should be in place to safeguard quality. Hence, fund providers, inventors, and clients have a constant responsibility to evaluate and scrutinize the performance of AI algorithms to ensure that AI technologies should not have any damaging influence on a particular patient. Inhibiting damage necessitates that usage of AI technologies does not consequence in any psychological or bodily harm. AI technologies that provide a judgement or cautionary that a specific cannot address because of lack of reasonable, reachable, or affordable healthcare should be prudently achieved.
- AI should be comprehensible or reasonable to designers, clients, and regulators. It can be achieved by enhancing the precision and explainability of AI technology. The mandate is provided that these should be explainable to the level of degree possible and as per the capacity of the person to whom the explanation is addressed.
- The data protection laws created commitments of explainability for automatic decision-making. Anyone who has raised the request is required to be informed in the most satisfactorily or customized manner. As these technologies are complicated, frustration may arise between the explainer and the person receiving the explanation. Hence, there is a possibility of a trade-off between full explainability of an algorithm (at the cost of accuracy) and improved accuracy (at the expense of explainability) (Fig. 8.4).
- The emphasis should be on human stakeholders to accomplish the tasks and foster responsibility. However, AI technologies perform tasks beneath suitable conditions. If somewhat went wrong in the application of an AI, there should be a response. Appropriate methods should be implemented to safeguard investigation and compensation for individuals unfavourably influenced by technology notified

Fig. 8.4 The relationship and possible fields of conflicts among the four notions of healthcare ethics and explicability [10]

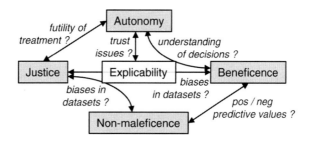

judgments. It should comprise effective treatments and recompense from governments and corporations that employ AI technologies for healthcare. Compensation, rehabilitation, restoration, penalties can be imposed along with the assurance of non-repetition. To evade dissemination of accountability, in which "everybody's problem becomes nobody's responsibility", or "collective responsibility" model, in which all the agents involved in the expansion and disposition of an AI technology are held accountable, can inspire all stakeholders to perform with honesty and diminish the damage. Here, the genuine intentions of stakeholders or their capability to manage an effect are not measured [7].

- Another emphasis is on inclusiveness, where healthcare is designed to promote the most significant possible, unbiased use, regardless of demographics, e.g. age, gender, income, ability, or other traits. The institutions (e.g. corporations, governing agencies, health organizations) should hire employees from disparate environments, ethnicities, and specialities to create, supervise, and implement AI. Involvement can also be enhanced by embracing open-source packages or making source codes openly obtainable. AI technologies should not be unfair. Prejudice is a threat to inclusiveness and fairness because it signifies a withdrawal, often illogical, from equal care. For instance, a system designed to diagnose cancerous skin lesions qualified with single skin colour data may not produce precise outcomes for patients with distinct skin colour, expanding the threat to their health.
- Receptiveness necessitates those engineers, designers, and clients constantly, thoroughly, and blatantly investigate an AI technology to ascertain whether it is reacting satisfactorily, aptly, and bestowing to communicated prospects and constraints in the perspective in which it is used. Therefore, recognizing a health need necessitates that institutions and governments react to that need and its philosophy with appropriate technologies to achieve the public interest in health protection and promotion. In case of technology is futile or provokes displeasure, the obligation to be quick to respond necessitates an institutional process to settle the problem, which may comprise ceasing use of the technology. Responsiveness also necessitates that AI technologies be steady with broader endeavours to stimulate health systems and ecological and workplace sustainability. Additionally, the methods should be devised to curtail their environmental trajectories and raise energy competence so that AI is coherent with society's efforts to reduce the impact of human beings on the earth's environment, ecosystems, and climate. Sustainability also obliges authorities and corporations to deliver anticipated disruptions to the workplace, including training of healthcare personnel to become accustomed to AI and probable job losses due to automatic systems for monotonous healthcare purposes and managerial tasks [8–11].

8.5 Summary

The digitalization of healthcare has posed many challenges with safeguarding ever-increasing volumes of hypersensitive and private information while sticking to state and national privacy and security guidelines. In today's scenario, AI requires enormous and disparate sorts of digital data but is susceptible to data infringements.

The fundamental issue will be protecting patient privacy and safeguarding their digital data; along with privacy and security, numerous legal and ethical questions will always arise. Consequently, it will be mandatory for healthcare advisors, AI designers, policymakers, data scientists, and various experts to recognize susceptibilities and contemplate pioneering and positive strategies to tackle them.

Additional byte

With the mordernization of healthcare, the HIPAA enforcement is much more stronger and violations of the rule may cost huge. The financial penalties for HIPAA violations are by the HIPAA Omnibus Rule.

Source https://www.hhs.gov/hipaa/for-professionals/compliance-enforcement/data/enforcement-highlights/index.html.

References

1. Vayena E, Dzenowagis J, Brownstein JS, Sheikh A (2018) Policy implications of big data in the health sector. Bull World Health Organ 96(1):66–68. https://doi.org/10.2471/blt.17.197426
2. Zhang D, Mishra S, Brynjolfsson E, Etchemendy J, Ganguli D, Grosz B, Lyons T, Manyika J, Niebles JC, Sellitto M, Shoham Y, Clark J, Perrault R (2021) The AI index 2021 annual report. Human-Centered AI Institute, Stanford University, AI Index Steering Committee, Stanford, CA
3. Gerke S, Minssen T, Cohen G (2020) Ethical and legal challenges of artificial intelligence-driven healthcare. Artif Intell Healthc 295–336.https://doi.org/10.1016/B978-0-12-818438-7.00012-5
4. Lo Piano S (2020) Ethical principles in machine learning and artificial intelligence: cases from the field and possible ways forward. Humanit Soc Sci Commun 7:9. https://doi.org/10.1057/s41599-020-0501-9
5. Braun M, Hummel P, Beck S, Dabrock P (2020) Primer on an ethics of AI-based decision support systems in the clinic. J Med Ethics. https://doi.org/10.1136/medethics-2019-105860. Epub ahead of print. PMID: 32245804
6. Biller-Andorno N, Ferrario A, Joebges S, Krones T, Massini F, Barth P, Arampatzis G, Krauthammer M (2021) AI support for ethical decision-making around resuscitation: proceed with care. J Med Ethics. https://doi.org/10.1136/medethics-2020-106786. Epub ahead of print. PMID: 33687916
7. Cath C (2018) Governing artificial intelligence: ethical, legal and technical opportunities and challenges. Philos Trans A Math Phys Eng Sci 376(2133):20180080. https://doi.org/10.1098/rsta.2018.0080. PMID: 30322996; PMCID: PMC6191666
8. Arnold MH (2021) Teasing out artificial intelligence in medicine: an ethical critique of artificial intelligence and machine learning in medicine. J Bioethical Inq 18(1):121–139. https://doi.org/10.1007/s11673-020-10080-1. Epub 2021 Jan 7. PMID: 33415596; PMCID: PMC7790358

 9. Gaur L, Solanki A, Wamba SF, Jhanjhi NZ Advanced AI techniques and applications in bioinformatics. CRC Press. https://doi.org/10.1201/9781003126164. ISBN: 978-0-367-64169-6 (hbk)
10. Beil M, Proft I, van Heerden D et al (2019) Ethical considerations about artificial intelligence for prognostication in intensive care. ICMx 7:70. https://doi.org/10.1186/s40635-019-0286-6
11. https://www.sanofi.com/en/about-us/our-stories/the-ethics-of-ai-in-healthcare. Accessed 12 July 2021
12. Rodrigues R (2020) Legal and human rights issues of AI: gaps, challenges and vulnerabilities. J Responsible Technol 4:100005. https://doi.org/10.1016/j.jrt.2020.100005. ISSN: 2666-6596

Printed in the United States
by Baker & Taylor Publisher Services